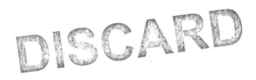

# HOW TO
# MAKE
# DISEASE
# DISAPPEAR

# HOW TO
# MAKE
# DISEASE
# DISAPPEAR

## DR. RANGAN CHATTERJEE

PHOTOGRAPHY BY SUSAN BELL

HarperOne
*An Imprint of* HarperCollins*Publishers*

HarperOne

HOW TO MAKE DISEASE DISAPPEAR. Copyright © 2018 by Rangan Chatterjee. All rights reserved. Printed in the United States of America. No part of this book may be used or reproduced in any manner whatsoever without written permission except in the case of brief quotations embodied in critical articles and reviews. For information, address HarperCollins Publishers, 195 Broadway, New York, NY 10007.

HarperCollins books may be purchased for educational, business, or sales promotional use. For information, please email the Special Markets Department at SPsales@harpercollins.com.

Originally published as *The Four Pillar Plan* in the United Kingdom in 2017 by Penguin Life, an imprint of Penguin Random House UK.

FIRST US EDITION

*Photography copyright © 2018 by Susan Bell*
*Illustrations copyright © 2018 by Son of Alan—Folio Art*

Library of Congress Cataloging-in-Publication Data has been applied for.

ISBN 978-0-06-284634-1

18 19 20 21 22  LSC  10 9 8 7 6 5 4 3 2 1

For my dad, you have influenced me
in more ways than you ever knew.
I wish you were still here.

# CONTENTS

# INTRODUCTION

We are sick and getting sicker. In the United States today, a new generation of children has been born that has a lower life expectancy than the generation before it. This is shocking and extraordinary. To understand why it's happening, we first have to grasp the terrible epidemic of chronic disease that's currently laying waste to millions.

Chronic diseases such as type 2 diabetes, high blood pressure, depression and dementia are today the nation's leading causes of death and disability. Half of all American adults currently suffer from a chronic disease, with one in four people suffering from two or more. Chronic disease is, by a wide margin, now the deadliest problem facing America. Despite the statistics and the suffering, so much confusion exists about what we can do in our own lives to protect ourselves and live long, healthy lives. I have seen this firsthand as I have lived and worked with many families.

The good news is that I can make these diseases disappear. That's right. This probably sounds like an extraordinary claim, but the reason I can make them disappear is that they're an illusion. These diseases are not the inevitable result of aging. They are not simply our genetic fate or our destiny. We do not have to suffer needlessly. The truth is these diseases don't really exist, at least not in the way we think they do.

To come to this conclusion, I first had to travel down a long, hard road. Seventeen years ago, I graduated from medical school full of enthusiasm and passion, ready to go out and help people. But I always felt there was something missing. I started off as a specialist and then became a generalist, as an MD, but I always had this nagging sense that I was just managing disease or simply suppressing

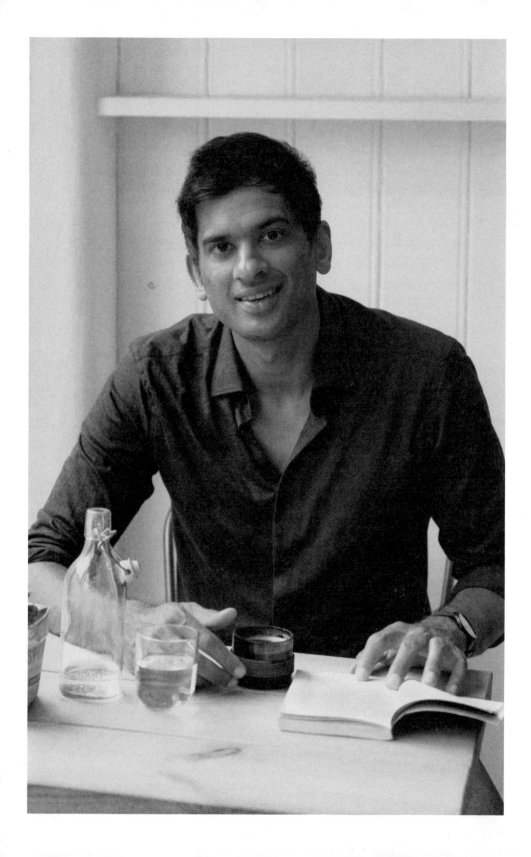

people's symptoms. And then on December 28, 2010, a turning point came. That was the day my son nearly died.

I was on a skiing vacation with my family in the stunning snowy landscape of Chamonix, France. My son had been a little phlegmy and quiet all day, but I wasn't too worried. It was just a cold and I felt sure it would pass without issue. That evening my wife, Vidh, sat on the sofa watching TV while I was in the kitchen. I was watching the kettle, waiting for the water to boil, when I heard her shout: "Rangan! He's not moving!" I rushed in. "He must be choking!" I said. "It's the phlegm." I lifted him out of Vidh's arms, turned him over and slapped him over the back in an attempt to clear his airway. But nothing happened. "Rangan, he's not choking," said Vidh. "We need to go to the hospital." My son's arms were stretched out, his body was rigid, his eyes stared vacantly.

After a panicked rush down a snowy road that almost ended in my turning the car over, we found ourselves standing in the resuscitation room of the emergency room of the tiny Les Hôpitaux du Pays du Mont-Blanc. As I watched the doctors take his temperature and try to get an intravenous line into his neck, I ran through the possibilities of what might be wrong with him. Was it epilepsy? Was it something more serious? I couldn't think. I felt numb. The truth was, I didn't have a clue. In that moment, I was no longer the doctor with nearly ten years' experience who'd graduated from the prestigious University of Edinburgh's medical school. I was a terrified dad.

Five long, agonizing hours later, the doctor came in to see us, waiting by our son's bed. "Dr. Chatterjee, we have an update," he said.

"What is it?" I asked.

"Dr. Chatterjee, your son's calcium levels are very low. In fact, he has almost no calcium in his body at all. He experienced a hypocalcemic convulsion. We're going to give him some intravenous calcium."

My reaction was utter confusion. How had this happened? What did it mean? But my confusion in that moment was nothing compared with the shock I felt when I did finally discover the root cause of what happened. It was an *entirely preventable* vitamin D deficiency. This was as unbelievable as it was serious. Untreated—especially in children—vitamin D deficiency can lead to painful and permanent damage including deformities to the bones, a condition known as rickets. I was devastated. And I swore that I would never allow anything like it to happen again.

The crisis of my son's illness forced me to ask some honest and uncomfortable questions. Why had I not been made sufficiently aware of vitamin and other nutritional deficiencies during my supposedly top-of-the-line medical training? And why wasn't that training proving more effective in my practice? As an MD, my days were filled with seeing patients with chronic conditions such as joint pain, headaches, type 2 diabetes, insomnia, depression, weight gain and fatigue. I hated to admit it, but the fact was, I reckoned I was helping maybe 20 percent of these people. The approach to consultations I'd been taught in medical school simply wasn't working. And if my medical training was failing me so badly for so many of my patients, what else could I do but embark on my own course of re-education?

And so began an incredible journey through many new worlds of knowledge that, I'm sad to say, the majority of doctors still have relatively little idea about. I immersed myself in research, especially around nutrition, movement science, stress reduction, ancestral health and functional medicine. I also came across research that allowed me to see afresh what I'd learned while completing my BSc honors degree in immunology, gaining valuable insight into the rapidly developing field of gut health and the microbiome. I started applying the science, first with my family and then with my patients. Do you know what happened? People started getting better—really better. I'd finally learned to resolve the root cause of their problems, rather than simply suppressing their symptoms.

What I'd learned, in a way that I hadn't fully grasped before, was that acute disease and chronic disease are entirely different things. Acute disease is something that, as doctors, we're pretty good at. It's relatively simple. You have something like pneumonia, a severe lung infection—so in your lung you have the overgrowth of some bugs, typically a type of bacteria. We identify the bacteria and we give you a treatment, typically an antibiotic that kills it. The bacteria die and, hey presto, you no longer have your pneumonia. The problem is, we apply that same thinking to chronic disease, and it simply doesn't work.

Chronic disease doesn't just happen like this. Chronic disease has many different causes. You don't just wake up some day suffering from one; by the time we give you the diagnosis, things have already been going wrong for a long, long time.

Let me tell you about one patient I met whom I found to be struggling with an all-too-common chronic disease. Thirty-five-year-old Mary was struggling with weight problems, joint problems, sleep problems and fatigue. I did some blood tests and diagnosed her with type 2 diabetes. This is one of the most harmful chronic diseases the world is currently facing. One in ten Americans currently has type 2 diabetes, and one in four has its precursor, pre-diabetes. The vast majority of sufferers don't even know they've got it. Between 1990 and 2013, rates of the disease shot up by an incredible 71 percent in the United States—one of the most dramatic increases of any nation. It currently costs the US alone more than $245 billion a year. Within thirty days of treating Mary, I'd made her diabetes disappear. Two years on, her "disease" is nowhere to be seen!

Most cases of type 2 diabetes are caused by something called insulin resistance. Insulin is a very important hormone, and one of its key functions is to keep your blood sugar tightly controlled in your body. Say you have a sugary bowl of cereal for breakfast. What happens is your blood sugar goes up, but your body releases a little bit of insulin and that helps it come back down to normal. The problem is, after years of dietary abuse with sugary foods, the insulin begins to lose its power. As you become more insulin resistant, you need more and more insulin to do the same job. You can think of it as a little like alcohol. The very first time you have a drink, what happens? Let's say some wine—one or two sips, or maybe half a glass—you feel tipsy, you feel a bit drunk. As you become a more seasoned and accustomed drinker, you need more and more alcohol to have the same effect, and that's what's going on with insulin. You need more and more insulin to have the same effect. When the insulin can no longer keep your sugar under control, despite its best efforts, we say you've got a disease, type 2 diabetes. However, things will have been going wrong in your body for many years before that.

But what causes insulin resistance in the first place? Actually, it's not just diet. It could also be that you're chronically stressed: work stress, emotional stress, physical stress. They can all raise levels of cortisol in your body, which raises your sugar, which in turn can contribute to insulin resistance. It could also be sleep deprivation. In some, losing one night of sleep can trigger as much insulin resistance as six months on a junk food diet. It could be age. The muscle mass we naturally lose as we get older can also cause insulin resistance. The problem is, there are many different causes of insulin resistance, and if we don't address *all* the causes for that particular patient, we'll never get rid of their disease. For Mary, I addressed the causes *for her,* and a few weeks later, she no longer had her "disease." That's right. In just a few weeks, no symptoms and no type 2 diabetes.

What about another chronic disease? As we live longer, many of us will have to face the devastating consequences of Alzheimer's. It's a heart-wrenching condition, and doctors and researchers are scrambling around trying to find the cure. It might surprise you to learn that one expert, Dr. Dale Bredesen, has successfully reversed early cognitive decline in some of his dementia patients. He's done that by working out what the various triggers have been in his individual patients and correcting them, reversing their symptoms. And which triggers is he looking at? He's examining many different factors including diet, stress levels and sleep quality as well as physical activity levels. Other prominent researchers in the field are applying similar strategies and are getting encouraging results.

Is this sounding a little bit familiar? These are some of the same causes of the insulin resistance that gives us type 2 diabetes. What if these, as well as many other seemingly separate chronic diseases, share common root causes? I believe they do.

The problem with the way we think about health and practice medicine is this: we forget that the human body is one big connected system. If it starts being treated poorly in one area, by bad diet or lack of sleep, problems can emerge in another part of it, often emerging as a so-called chronic disease. Then, if a patient presents with depression, we'll prescribe an antidepressant. But depression can just as easily be driven by poor diet or high stress levels—or, even more likely, *both*. It's the same with a condition like eczema. Doctors all too often just prescribe a steroid cream for the rash, but the rash is only a symptom. There's very little awareness that the *causes* of eczema are many, and that it may be triggered by an overreactive immune system that may itself be caused by food choices or abnormalities with gut bacteria. A human being is a highly evolved biological mechanism that's completely, what I call "massively," interconnected. Because of this, a symptom in one domain might actually have a cause way upstream, in an area of the body that our medical training just doesn't tell us to look in.

Because everything in our bodies affects, to a greater or lesser degree, pretty much everything else, we need to take a much more global view of treatment, one that considers every aspect of the way the patient is living their life. How are they sleeping? How are they eating? Do they sit behind a desk for hours a day not moving? Are they constantly on their phones? I call this the "threshold effect." The massively connected system that is in the human body can deal with multiple insults in various places—up to a point. And then the system breaks down, often with a new problem in some distant part

*"The benefits will happen immediately and the results last a lifetime. This is a radical health journey that's designed for everyone."*

of the system. That point at which it breaks down is our own, unique, personal threshold. When talking to patients, I liken it to juggling. We can often juggle one ball, two balls, even three or four. But when we throw that fifth one in, *all* the balls fall down. We get sick. That sickness might manifest as a skin complaint or a blood sugar problem or a mood disorder or difficulty sleeping. These complaints are all downstream signals that things—usually more than one—are going wrong upstream. Unlike many other doctors, I start upstream, not down.

I'm not a scientist, I'm a doctor, and they are not the same things at all. My job is to read the science, then interpret it in the context of the patient who's with me. The science doesn't tell me everything I need to know. Something essential also comes from hearing a patient's individual story. I believe the most skilled and effective healers are the ones who listen. I also believe that medicine is art *and* science. It's the blending of the two. We too often forget this and are then surprised by all the discrepancies there are between what lab trials show and what we find happening in real life. Science doesn't do everything. I don't give two hoots if there's a study to show reducing our exposure to social media makes us less stressed. You can get data to show black is white and white is black. You can manipulate trials and data to say what you want. What I'm giving you is my seventeen years of experience as an MD seeing tens of thousands of patients, but this is my belief. It's based on science, but it's also based on my own experience. If you disagree with me, I'm OK with that. I believe my decade and a half of practice qualifies me to make simple recommendations that, as long as they do no harm, don't need to wait for all the science to catch up. By practicing this way, I've managed to avoid sending hundreds of patients down the road of medicalization, and cured many hundreds more.

I have written this book to provide a simple, actionable plan to help you take control of your health. There's nothing in here that's got any downside. No confusion. No bad science. Just practical solutions, based on seventeen years of clinical experience, to help disease disappear. The benefits will happen immediately and the results last a lifetime. This is a radical health journey that's designed for everyone. The worst thing that's going to happen (and I don't think it will) is you end up feeling the same. The best? You'll completely transform your life—and have a lot more of it to live.

The tools in this book may seem simple and even somehow "unmedical," but don't be fooled—they will have a profound impact on your biology. They'll make a difference—to your hormones, to your inflammatory cytokines, to the level of reactive oxygen species in your blood, and on and on. These are not soft interventions. This is not soft medicine. This is real medicine that is targeted especially to our unprecedented epidemic of lifestyle illnesses; you can't expect to avoid the deadly diseases that have taken so many millions of lives if you continue living without it.

Let's go beyond the typical health advice we've been reading about for so long—beyond the fad diets and quick-fix programs. We have overcomplicated health—and I want to simplify it. This book is the practical, achievable approach you have been waiting for. Everything you need to know about starting or continuing a radical health journey is in these pages. Join me as we make disease disappear.

# HOW TO USE THIS BOOK

There are four main elements, or pillars, to the plan. The aim of the book is to examine and improve the manner in which you Relax, Eat, Move and Sleep. For each pillar I have set out five ways you might do this, summarized in the opposite table. The idea is to create balance across all the pillars—it is not about perfection in each individual one.

I would much rather you score 2 in every pillar, giving you a total score of 8, rather than 5 out of 5 in two separate pillars, giving you a higher score of 10. The numerical score might be less but the balance is greater, and this is the real point of the book. Achieving balance is what will lead to the biggest improvements and, most importantly, the sustainable ones. This is designed to be a whole-life plan rather than a quick-fix gimmick.

For most of my patients, most of the time, doing 3 in each pillar, resulting in a total score of 12, seems to be about right. It is simply impossible, however, for me to say what will be the right amount for you. Some of you will need to do more, some can get away with less.

It is possible, though, to take each pillar in isolation. You may already feel, for example, that your diet and exercise are already dialed in, whereas your sleep needs a bit more attention. If this is the case, feel free to go straight to that individual pillar and start there. You do not need to go through the book in sequential order if you don't want to. I want you to personalize this book, so it suits your own life.

Give equal priority to every pillar, and proceed at a pace that is comfortable for you.

## RELAX

Fifteen minutes of me-time every day ✓

Weekly screen-free Sabbath ✓

Keep a gratitude journal ✓

A daily practice of stillness ✓

Eat one meal per day around a table— without an e-device ✓

## EAT

De-normalize sugar (and retrain your taste buds) ✓

Eat five different vegetables every day ✓

Eat your food within a twelve-hour window ✓

Drink eight glasses of water per day ✓

Unprocess your diet by avoiding food products with more than five ingredients ✓

## MOVE

Walk 10,000 steps per day ✓

Twice a week, do a form of strength training ✓

Twice a week, do a form of high-intensity interval training ✓

Daily movement snacks ✓

Daily glute exercises to help wake them up ✓

## SLEEP

Create an environment of absolute darkness ✓

Spend at least twenty minutes outside every morning ✓

Create a bedtime routine ✓

Manage your commotion ✓

Enjoy your caffeine before noon ✓

# RELAX

What I'm about to say probably sounds far-fetched, but here it is. The health problems of the majority of patients I see—yes, the *majority*—are driven entirely by their lifestyle. It's not cuts or bruises or bacteria or a fungus or a virus or some tumor or hereditary disorder that's the source of their pain, but the way they're choosing to live. Their conditions are very often exacerbated by the fact that they're super busy. They wake up fully stressed, rush to get the kids ready, do the school run, come back, try to juggle their jobs and their home life. On top of that, they might have other family members who require care and attention. From the moment they open their eyes, it's all go, go, go. Then, when their kids are finally in bed, they're straight into their emails or social media. At no point in the day are they just chilling out, or even alone. Everything they do is for someone else. When I mention this in my office, they roll their eyes, telling me, "But I just don't have time for me." To which I reply, "Well that, right there, is your problem."

# GIVE YOURSELF PERMISSION TO RELAX

I never thought that, as a doctor, I'd have to give anyone permission to do anything. I see my patients as adults who can make their own decisions. But daily experience has taught me that, when it comes to relaxation, a surprising number of people don't get any. So here I am, giving you doctor's orders: I want you to give daily relaxation as high a priority as food, movement and sleep. I think our lack of routine switch-off time is one of the most pressing issues in modern society. For your health, it could hardly be more critical.

In this Relax pillar, as in the other three, you'll find five different interventions. While you are reading through them, start to think about which ones resonate the most, and which ones you might be able to introduce into your life right away. I would love you to adopt at least three, but if that seems too daunting, build up to it by taking on one at a time. I'm the type who's always desperate to jump in and attempt the lot, but we're all different, and it's really important that you find your own pace. It really doesn't matter *how* you get there, as long as you get there.

The Relax pillar is the one I struggle with the most. However, despite many challenges along the way, I've seen the benefits in my own life. I've also seen it in my practice. Potential gains include:

- Weight loss
- Improved resilience
- Reduced feelings of stress
- Improved ability to cope
- More balanced outlook
- Less road rage
- Improved ability to sleep
- More restorative sleep
- Better concentration

There is a reason why I've started this book with the Relax pillar. It's the one that most often gets ignored, both by the public and also by the plethora of quick-fix health books that are out there. Which intervention should you start with? I genuinely don't believe there's much between them but, if you made me choose, the two I would prioritize are the first—carving out some me-time every single day—and the fourth—a daily practice of stillness. The benefits are not only immense but also can be rapid, which will help you engage with the others.

# 1. ME-TIME EVERY DAY

*Every day, for at least fifteen minutes, be selfish,*
*and enjoy some time for you.*

For at least fifteen minutes, every day, and more if possible, stop everything and be utterly selfish. Stop treating "relaxation" as something that you do—or, more likely, don't do—when everything else has been dealt with. *Choose* to relax. Make it a triple-underlined part of your schedule. Set an alarm. What will you do? Will you visit a local cafe, buy a coffee and indulge in a trashy magazine? Will you sit in a room with the lights off, listening to your favorite piece of music? Will you enjoy a relaxing bath? It's entirely up to you. But there are three rules. Firstly, it must be something unashamedly for you and you alone. Secondly, it must not be an activity that involves your smartphone, tablet or computer. Thirdly, you're not allowed to feel guilty about it.

## CORTISOL SURGE

Had you told me this a few years ago, I wouldn't have believed it, but simply setting aside little moments every day can make a massive difference to your health. There are many reasons why these breaks make a difference, but a principal one is that they can help us to switch off our overactive stress response. Now, we all have cortisol in our bodies, and we all need it. Cortisol is a hormone, and a hormone is a chemical messenger. When we feel hungry, satiated, aroused, angry and so on, it's because particular hormones are surging around our bloodstreams. Cortisol has been identified as one of our principal stress-response hormones. Hormone levels tend to spike and fall at different times of the day, in natural cycles, and also rise and fall in response to the things that are happening to us. Our cortisol level surges when we're stressed.

Contrary to popular belief, stress isn't necessarily bad for us. We've evolved to experience stress for all sorts of good reasons. An onrush of stress primes our minds and bodies to tackle a sudden problem head-on. But we're designed to experience stress in short bursts. When we endure it for a sustained period, it becomes a problem. To find out why this is, we must cast our view back hundreds of thousands of years. Humans are the product of an extremely gradual process of evolution that took place over many millennia. Our bodies and brains have been specialized, not for modern living in towns and cities, but for existence in roaming hunter-gatherer groups of no more than 150 people. Because this kind of evolution occurs so slowly, our ancient systems haven't caught up with twenty-first-century life. Our machinery for responding to and dealing with stress is still largely prehistoric. And that mismatch between the ancient biological technology we have in our bodies and the complex, ultra-modern lives we're living can have some pretty nasty effects.

**NORMAL CORTISOL RHYTHM THROUGHOUT THE DAY**

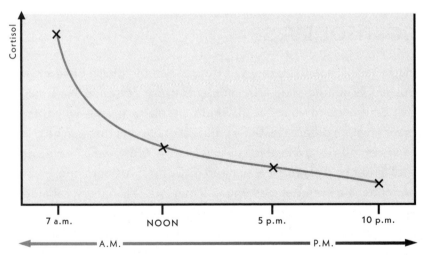

    HOW TO MAKE DISEASE DISAPPEAR

Imagine what kind of stresses our bodies were designed to cope with all those years ago. If we were attacked by a lion, say, that experience would be terrifying but it would also be short lived. Either we'd have run away and escaped, or killed the lion, and the danger would have passed, or we'd have been killed. That's the kind of event our stress equipment has been built to deal with. Our autonomic nervous system is a bodily network around which signals and instructions are transmitted, and there are two parts to it, the sympathetic system and the parasympathetic. Cortisol works by activating our sympathetic nervous system. This is our fight-or-flight response. And what I'm seeing in my practice is that people are *constantly* in fight-or-flight mode. They're spending their days with their cortisol levels continuously ramped right up, their sympathetic nervous systems activated. They're not being attacked by a lion, they're being attacked by their life.

## CORTISOL STEAL

This is harmful for a number of reasons. Firstly, there's something called the "cortisol steal." All the hormones in your body are made from the same basic stuff, which is called LDL cholesterol. We naturally have a limited supply of LDL cholesterol and, when things are working well, it all gets portioned off nicely, so there's enough to go around—enough to make your estrogen, your progesterone, your testosterone—and also your cortisol. But what happens when you're in one of these long-term states of stress is that cortisol steals the other hormones' LDL cholesterol. Because it thinks you're under attack, and in a state of crisis, your body prioritizes the generation of cortisol. It thinks you need it to cope with the drama and just makes more and more of it. That upsets the finely tuned balance of hormones in your body.

# THE TWO PARTS OF THE
# AUTONOMIC NERVOUS SYSTEM

Our autonomic nervous system regulates our automatic processes—the things we do without consciously thinking, like breathing and digestion.

One branch of this system, the sympathetic nervous system, causes the body to release stress-response hormones such as noradrenaline and cortisol. It causes your heart rate to quicken, your lung tubes to widen, your muscles to contract, and your pupils to dilate, and it switches off digestion. It helps divert energy away from processes in our body such as digestion that are not necessary for our survival. It helps us release energy from our muscles and lowers immune system function. In the short term this helps us deal with the stress, but if activated long term this response can become problematic.

In the modern world, this fight-or-flight system activates when we're rushing to meet a deadline, getting stressed on our commute, leaving late for the school run or putting ourselves through a tough workout. This response can be managed, as long as we take steps to balance it out with rest and relaxation.

This rest and relaxation involves the other branch of our nervous system, which is the parasympathetic. It works at a much slower rate than the sympathetic branch. When it's activated our saliva production increases, digestive enzymes are released, our heart rate drops and our muscles relax. It allows us to digest food appropriately, destress and sleep soundly.

To help manage the stress of modern life we should be encouraging the activation of the parasympathetic nervous system—all five interventions in the Relax pillar will help you do just that.

This leads to a wide variety of problems. Clinicians know we're currently seeing an increase in numbers of men with low testosterone. This impacts things like sex drive, muscular strength, energy levels and even risk of chronic disease, and testosterone prescriptions now cost the NHS (National Health Service, the UK's healthcare system) something like £20 million (about $27.6 million) per year. I'm convinced the underlying problem in many of these cases is stress, leading to overproduction of cortisol at the expense of other hormones, of which testosterone is just one.

But it's not just the cortisol steal we need to be concerned about. When we're constantly stressed, our bodies respond as if we're under attack, going into a kind of emergency mode and diverting resources to the processes most necessary for survival. To take just one example, digestion switches off. When you're dealing with a lion flying at your head, the efficient processing of lunch is just an unnecessary diversion. A more pressing need is the generation of instant energy in your bloodstream. In the short term this is great, but when this becomes long term it creates a problem. It can lead to weight gain and sleep disruption and exhausts the immune system. Remember, all of this is happening because the body thinks it's under attack all day. While there are an infinite number of stressors in our environment, there's only one main stress response. Your body can't tell the difference between emotional stress, physical stress and nutritional stress. It can't tell the difference between the stress of missing a mortgage payment or the stress you feel when someone's been rude to you on Facebook. To your system, it's all just a lion flying at your head and it reacts in the same way in every case.

## IMPACT ON YOUR DIGESTIVE SYSTEM

You know when you get that mid-morning hunger surge? You've had your bowl of sugar-coated cereal, your blood sugar's gone up, then mid-morning it's crashed. You're starving. You're shaky. You need something to eat. When your blood sugar falls suddenly like this, that's another stressor, another lion at your head. It can send your cortisol and adrenaline soaring. So even something as simple as choosing the wrong breakfast can tip your body into this emergency state. Then what happens? Not only are you likely to go hunting in your fridge or cookie jar for some more bad food, your digestion is suppressed, so it's a double hit on the weight gain. This is another example of why it's crucial that we view the body as a massively connected system. One potential cause—in this case, a sugary breakfast—can have multiple effects, including stress, the cortisol steal and weight gain.

## IMPACT ON YOUR IMMUNE SYSTEM

But that's not all. When your body thinks it's under attack, it puts your immune system into an emergency state. This makes perfect sense from an evolutionary perspective. Imagine if you managed to survive that lion attack by fighting it off. It's likely you'd be left with cuts that were prone to infection—the animal would've had nasty bugs in its claws or saliva and your wounds would pick up dirt from your environment. This is why your immune system needs to go into a peak state. We call this heightened immune response "inflammation" and, again, we're not supposed to be in this state for an extended period of time. Chronic inflammation (in medical parlance, any nasty condition that hangs around for too long is referred to as "chronic") underpins pretty much every single degenerative disease that we have, including heart attacks, strokes and even Alzheimer's disease.

A 2016 paper published by researchers at King's College London highlighted just one of the ways inflammation can have a surprising impact on the massively connected body. They showed a remarkable link between inflammation and depression. The scientists suggested we can predict which patients suffering from depression will respond to conventional antidepressants by giving them blood tests that show their levels of inflammation. Crucially, they found that patients with high degrees of inflammation do not respond to conventional antidepressants. The results confirm what other scientific research has been suggesting for years—that depression itself can be a symptom of biological changes in the body that are driven by inflammation. This is why antidepressants don't work for these patients. If your problem is not in your brain—if it's actually inflammation in your body—what's the point in giving you a drug that's going to tweak something in your head?

Think about how astonishing this is. If someone is depressed, the textbook medicine approach points our clinical gaze at possible struggles they're having in their life, or past traumas, or perhaps even chemical problems in their brain. But the root cause might just as easily be inflammation that's caused by having too much cortisol charging about their system, for too long. This is how healthcare needs to evolve—into an era of progressive medicine characterized by the growing awareness that the name of a disease can often tell us very little about the actual cause. "Depression" is simply a name we give to a collection of symptoms—the word itself doesn't tell us anything about the root of the problem.

Understanding all this is increasingly transforming the way I practice medicine. Recently I was consulted by Miranda, a fifty-two-year-old whom I hadn't seen for about six months. She had been following all my advice but now had seemed to plateau, and was not improving any further. I spent a long time chatting with her to try to figure out why. As we got into her story, it became clear that she had no time for herself at all. She was always on the go and she never stopped.

When I put this to her, she said, "Family life is just stressful." I tested her saliva. As I expected, her cortisol levels were through the roof. I kicked myself for not going down this path sooner. Stress is now a critical line of investigation I pursue in relation to a huge array of complaints.

## STRESS AND MENOPAUSE

I've treated menopausal difficulties in women by helping them deal more effectively with their stress levels. These women have a problem with their hormones, namely estrogen and progesterone. The textbook medicine approach often results in doctors prescribing a course of hormone replacement therapy (HRT), which can comprise various combinations of these female hormones. Not only is HRT a cost burden on the patient and the healthcare system, it can also have some unpleasant side-effects, including bloating, swelling, nausea, cramps and even vaginal bleeding. There are also ongoing concerns about possible increased risks of ovarian cancer, breast cancer and blood clots.

There's no doubt that HRT often works, but is it always necessary? If the patient is stressed, most of her body's LDL cholesterol is likely going straight into making cortisol. This means there's less of it left to make estrogen and progesterone. HRT deals with the symptom, but why not go to the root cause instead? Normalizing cortisol levels— whether through meditation (see page 42) or from sectioning off some daily me-time, or even from switching to a whole-food diet (which helps reduce the nutritional stress caused by low-quality foods)—very often alleviates menopausal symptoms entirely.

## STRESS AND THE GUT

Using these principles, I once treated a forty-year-old woman who had a bad case of Crohn's disease. Crohn's is a nasty bowel complaint and she'd been getting painful stomach cramps and kept needing to go to the bathroom. Nothing seemed to be helping her and she'd reached the point where she was losing patience with her specialist. Eventually, she came in to see me. I made some changes to her diet that helped for a while, but she quickly plateaued. I couldn't understand why this was, so I decided to delve deeper. I soon realized she literally had nothing in her daily life for herself. Everything was to do with her kids and her husband. She was going at full speed all the time, never putting herself first. "Are there any other medications I should be trying?" she asked. "What else should I do with my diet?"

---

### CYTOKINES

Cytokines are proteins released by the immune system. They work as messengers, taking the information being put out by the immune system around the body. They are essential to immune system function and are involved with coordinating the initiation, maintenance and resolution of all immune responses. Maintaining a delicate balance in the level of these communicators is vital for health.

The immune system releases cytokines in response not only to infections and traumatic accidents but also to triggers such as stress, food and exercise.

Their release is tightly regulated as their impact can be severe: some of them cause inflammation while others have the opposite effect. Some, including interleukin 6, can serve both functions in different situations.

---

"You know what?" I said. "I'm going to try something completely different. I'm going to give you another appointment in a month. In the meantime, here's what I want you to do." I took out my notepad and wrote a list of three things. "Two fifteen-minute periods for you per day. A walk every morning. And find something to do, at least twice a week, that you love and that you do just for you."

After falling out with her specialist, this was the last thing she wanted to hear. I could see it written all over her face—she thought I was reverting to soft, woolly, paternalistic medicine. Perhaps she even felt patronized. She had a serious illness and she expected serious medicine. "And what about supplements?" she asked me crossly. "What about medication?"

"That's it," I said. "That's all I want you to do." I pushed the note toward her. "This is your prescription."

Now, I knew this patient very well. Despite her suspicions, she trusted me and I was hopeful that she'd at least give it a chance. When she came back four weeks later, I was delighted. She told me she'd joined a salsa class, which was something she'd been thinking about for years but had never done because she didn't think she had time. She'd also started going out for a walk in the mornings. She'd spent time in her living room, leaving her phone and laptop on the kitchen counter, just sitting and listening to music for fifteen minutes. We completed a medical symptom questionnaire, which is designed to measure objectively the effects of illness with questions such as how often she had stomach cramps or bowel movements. Even I was astonished to find her Crohn's symptoms had reduced by 50 percent. This kind of reduction in a four-week time frame, for a condition as complex and serious as Crohn's, is simply incredible.

What, to the outside observer, might be even more surprising is that the symptoms of Crohn's are located in the gut and none of the interventions I gave her seemed to have anything to do with that part of her body. But I know that if cortisol is up, it won't just affect how calm you're feeling, it will affect your gut function. Not only that but your inflammation markers go up, and the way your cytokines, which are chemicals that send messages within the immune system, behave changes. What does all this tell us? It tells us that the body is massively connected. Although she had a gut problem, her non-switching-off problem was making it worse. Of course, I'm not saying this will work for every Crohn's patient. There's simply no trial that says that this is *the* way to treat it—and nor is there likely to be. But that's not because interventions like this don't work. It's because everyone who has Crohn's is different.

I feel strongly that, as a doctor, I should try to follow my own advice and, by and large, I do. One of my patients, a firefighter, once told me the only reason he was going to do as I suggested was that I was the first doctor he'd seen who actually practiced what he preached.

I'll be honest, though—in the past, I have struggled to find time for me. But not anymore: I have built me-time into my daily routine. At my last practice, midway through the morning I allowed time for a fifteen-minute walk. Reception knew not to book anyone in between 10:15 and 10:30 a.m. Even if there were patients waiting I would still stop everything and go for a stroll. At first my manager wasn't at all happy—"Why is he doing this when he ought to be seeing patients?"—but she quickly realized that I would still see as many patients as anyone else, if not more.

Recently, I have re-engaged with cooking while having a favorite CD on—it is amazing how relaxing this can be. What can you do to give you your daily dose?

# EXAMPLES OF PHONE-FREE ME-TIME YOU MIGHT CONSIDER

| | | |
|---|---|---|
| Having a bath ✓ | Playing music ✓ |
| Going for a walk ✓ | Gardening ✓ |
| Sitting in a cafe having a drink ✓ | Cooking with your favorite album playing, or in silence ✓ |
| Sitting on a park bench relaxing ✓ | Painting ✓ |
| Reading a magazine ✓ | Dancing ✓ |
| Reading a book ✓ | Fifteen minutes of yoga or tai chi ✓ |
| Singing ✓ | Relaxing at home, with or without music ✓ |

You can also bring in components of your daily stillness practice (see page 42).

*I prioritize me-time. It's scheduled into my daily timetable. In today's world there's always something else to do—an email to send, a Facebook feed to scroll, a tweet to reply to. It's never-ending. That's why you need to make a proactive decision to prioritize that time.*

One of my recent patients, forty-four-year-old Suzanne, was busy juggling motherhood and a part-time job. When she told me she didn't have time for herself, I said to her, "Suzanne, after you've dropped the kids off, you go straight to the shops, back home, straight to emails and then you're go-go-go all day until it is time to pick them up. What would happen if your car broke down? You'd stop for an hour or so while you waited for the breakdown service. That would enforce your switch-off time. You'd still get everything done afterward, wouldn't you?" This resonated with her. She made it a rule every day after the kids were dropped off to go for a phone-free fifteen-minute walk, rain or shine. Six weeks later, she felt like a different person. She was less stressed throughout the day, and, counterintuitively, actually became *more* productive and got more things done. This tiny change had a huge impact.

Just by making space for yourself for fifteen minutes per day, as Suzanne did, you can help normalize your cortisol levels. Your body will be reminded what it's like not to feel under attack. I contend that modern living, even if it's something as simple and common as your email inbox overflowing, is stressful. *I* find it stressful. And what's the downside, in our busy culture, of actually trying this? There's none whatsoever. Ironically it's the people who say they don't have time for these interventions who need to do them the most.

# 2. THE SCREEN-FREE SABBATH

*Every Sunday, turn off your screens and live your day offline.*

It was a typically hectic day at my Oldham practice, at the end of a Monday afternoon, and I was running late. In the NHS, we're allotted ten minutes for each patient and it's easy to find your appointments running into each other. Your only hope for getting back on track is to luck into seeing a few people you can deal with speedily. This is what I was hoping would happen last summer when a sixteen-year-old named Devon came in, accompanied by his mom. But the moment they sat down, I realized this would be anything but a quick one. "Dr. Chatterjee," said the mother, struggling slightly to get the words out. "On Saturday night, Devon cut his wrists with a knife."

"On purpose?" I asked.

"On purpose," she nodded. "I had to take him to A&E [the emergency room]. The psychiatrist there said we should see you for antidepressants. We're here for the prescription."

It would've taken thirty seconds to write them a note for Prozac and send them on their way. But something stopped me. We started chatting and slowly Devon began to open up. I knew I had patients who were being delayed, but I also knew I couldn't do this boy a disservice. I needed to understand, why would a sixteen-year-old boy, from a seemingly well-balanced family, start self-harming out of nowhere?

As I probed, I discovered that he felt like a misfit at school, partly because of his hobbies and partly because of his appearance. I started asking him about social media usage.

"Do you go on it quite a lot?"

"I go on it loads," he grinned.

"Do you use it in bed at night?'

"Yeah, I'll go on Facebook, I'll be texting."

"Look," I said, "I'm wondering whether your use of social media is contributing to this in a small way." His face fell and his mother looked dubious. "Would you consider reducing it?"

"Why?" he said.

"I'm not sure it's helping your mental health. Your self-harming is a symptom. I want to find out what's causing it. An hour before bed, how about if you just switch your phone off? Do you think you could do that?"

"Errm," he said.

"I'll tell you what. Why don't you give it a go for a week? If you're still feeling the same, I'll write you that script."

I imagine that some of you may have been getting palpitations just from reading the title of this chapter. I know how you feel. I used to feel that way too. It's not that I'm against social media or the internet—not all. But I am seeing a huge rise in problems that stem from their use. This is hardly surprising, given their rapid ascent and infiltration into every aspect of our lives. It's now thought that there are more mobile devices on the planet than people—truly remarkable. Some of us—me included—can find it hard to leave our e-devices alone for more than ten minutes. If I'm playing with my kids on a Sunday and my phone's nearby, there's a constant nagging impulse to look at it. And I know for a fact that I am not the only one. We're encouraged to keep on checking our feeds, to see how many likes or followers we have, or to update ourselves on the

*"Studies suggest that humans spend as much as 40 percent of our speech time informing others about our own subjective experiences. It's believed that doing this fires up neural pathways associated with reward and activates addiction centers in the brain such as the nucleus accumbens."*

latest gossip. We have even started looking at our work emails on our days off. This contributes to the wider problem, one that's become exponentially more problematic since the introduction of smartphones. We are all finding it harder to switch off. When we open our eyes in the morning, instead of letting our bodies gradually awaken we're straight onto Twitter or Facebook or Snapchat, or whatever the latest social platform is, letting this constant stream of noise into our brains. And this noise is a huge problem. Five years ago, I was convinced that the root cause of most of the complaints I saw in my practice was poor diet. Now I'm convinced it's stress.

# SMARTPHONE ADDICTION

There's quite a bit of controversy out there about whether or not we can, in a truly clinical sense, say that the use of smartphones can be addictive. But real-world experience has left me in little doubt. One 2014 study of 2,000 people in the UK painted a disturbing portrait of the average user. We check our phones 221 times a day, starting at around 7:31 a.m., when we'll look at Facebook, read the news and check the weather before we've even gotten out of bed. By the time we go to sleep, we'll have spent three hours and sixteen minutes on our device. An even more alarming statistic from the US estimates that the average user touches their phone 2,617 times per day.

A large part of why these numbers are so ridiculously high is the fact that we're now constantly contactable, and subject to a ceaseless barrage of emails, calls and texts. But what's also happened, in the last ten or so years, is the beginning of an unhealthy "selfie" culture that feeds our phone addiction even more. Studies suggest that humans spend as much as 40 percent of our speech time informing others about our own subjective experiences. It's believed that doing this fires up neural pathways associated with reward and activates addiction centers in the brain such as the nucleus accumbens. It's easy to see how a few selfies with mindless updates on Facebook, Instagram and Snapchat can start to create a feedback loop in your brain where you crave more and more of the same. My experience has been that, just like many drugs, the more you use your smartphone, the more addicted you become.

We've evolved to enjoy social validation. We're highly social creatures. Just as the company making Snickers bars takes advantage of the fact we've evolved to love sweetness, so social media takes advantage of the fact we've evolved to crave the approval of others.

But, just like the 6.75 teaspoons of sugar you'll find in a Snickers bar, we were never designed to have so much of it. When the massively connected human machine was evolving, we expected to have sugar now and again, especially in the summer. This is what that machine still expects. It's what it was designed for. We also used to have the tribe applauding us once every now and then when we did something truly selfless or brave. But we now live in an age when we can have all these things all the time. We're overusing all our built-in evolutionary mechanisms. And you'd have to be naive to think there aren't going to be consequences.

An additional problem is what psychologists who study social media are now describing as "perfectionist presentation." People don't tend to post on the bad parts of their day, they tend to focus on the good stuff. This creates a false reality in which it can seem like everyone else is much more successful, and enjoying a much better life, than we are. We all tend to compare our lives to other people's and judge ourselves accordingly. These are automatic processes. We can't help it. In vulnerable adolescents, this can be an easy road to stress and depression. It can be just as harmful in adults.

# RESET YOUR RELATIONSHIP

One way in which you can start to reset your relationship with electronic media is by altering how you use your smartphone. I have tried this over the past eighteen months and immediately felt the benefits. Taking notifications off your phone is a great place to start. All your apps are still there and functioning, but every time someone likes an Instagram comment you've liked, or checks your profile on LinkedIn, you don't get a notification. You could extend this further by turning off the auto-sync on your email inbox. Now you have to physically request your email inbox to refresh.

I used to be addicted to the sight of a new notification on the screen of my phone. Now I don't see them. I can pick my phone up to make a call, blissfully unaware that I have ten new emails waiting for me. This may not sound like much in isolation, but when you think about how many times we look at our phones every day, this adds up to a lot of time. You could even try introducing a "device box" at home into which everyone in your household has to drop their phone before meals. The possibilities are endless and it is simply impossible for me to say what will end up working for you in the context of your own life. What helps pretty much everyone, however, is making some kind of change, no matter how small. Remember, every time you hear a notification or the ping of a new email you activate reward signals in your brain that leave you craving more.

What I hear again and again from my patients is that they had no idea how great an impact their e-device was having on their lives. There's no downtime when you have a smartphone in your pocket. How often do you go out for dinner and you're with your partner or best friend, but you're really not with them? How many times have you felt a "phantom phone buzz" in your pocket? What's *that* about?

and produce various by-products including short-chain fatty acids, or SCFAs. These SCFAs, including the most studied one, butyrate, are anti-inflammatory. This means that they help bring down the inflammation whose harmful effects—including heart disease, stroke, Alzheimer's disease—we first heard about in the Relax pillar when discussing the importance of me-time and communal meal-times. This is just a tiny part of that picture and it hopefully shows why simply thinking about diet in terms of calories, carbs and fat is so limiting.

that the presence of this bug is associated with better weight control, insulin sensitivity and much more. Obese people tend to have less Akkermansia muciniphila than lean people. If we don't have enough of it we are at greater risk of becoming obese or diabetic. Remarkably, after weight loss surgery people's Akkermansia muciniphila levels increase. While it's very hard to tease out cause and effect, it does appear that there is a compelling link between this particular gut bug and maintaining a healthy weight.

The gut has a protective lining of mucus that Akkermansia muciniphila feeds on, but it also feeds on:

- onions
- garlic
- leeks
- artichokes

- yams
- agave
- bananas
- brussels sprouts

- okra
- cauliflower
- broccoli
- chicory root

Akkermansia muciniphila adores these foods and will expand its numbers if fed accordingly. Fasting also leads to an increase in Akkermansia muciniphila, which is the subject of the next intervention.

# BUILDING UP YOUR IMMUNE SYSTEM

Because the body is so interconnected, by feeding the microbiome we're also strengthening other parts of it, such as our immune system. It's common to think of the immune system as something that is there simply to protect us from airborne bacteria and viruses and prevent coughs and colds. While that's true, 70 percent of our immune system activity takes place in and around our gut. This makes perfect sense, of course, because our gut is one of the key interfaces between the external world and our bodies. According to one study, there are actually more immune reactions in your gut, over the course of one day, than in the rest of your body in your entire lifetime. This seems extraordinary until you remember that everything you put into your mouth is a foreign body.

Specialized cells living in and around the gut lining use microscopic antennae to sample our food and check everything that passes through it. This information gathering, along with other signals, allows the immune system to make an active decision whether to let it in willingly or whether to react against it. If it reacts against it, the responses all involve the generation of inflammation and we can suffer myriad symptoms such as skin rashes, mood problems and joint pain. This happens because the system has become unruly and hypersensitive. You can think of the immune system as an army that's there to protect you from malevolent invaders. In a country that's in chaos, the army is out of control, overreacting and attacking everyone and everything—this is chronic inflammation. Eating certain foods can trigger the sending out of chemicals called cytokines that act as messengers, transmitting signals to the system that our bodies are under attack. But eating the right kind of foods can help bring that army back under control. It can give it order and discipline, making it more likely to attack only enemy targets and with a proportionate level of force.

Remember how good we said broccoli was as a means of feeding our microbiome? It also has a beneficial impact on our immune system. Before it even reaches the colon, where the gut bugs live, it arrives in the small intestine. On your small intestine you've got a kind of lock that will only take a particular key. This lock is called the aryl hydrocarbon receptor, or AHR. Certain vegetables—especially the cruciferous ones, such as cauliflower, broccoli, cabbage—have the correct key for the AHR lock. Bits of that broccoli will go into that AHR lock. When this happens, we get rewarded with a proliferation of what are called intraepithelial lymphocytes. These are fantastic, because they discipline your immune system. They calm it down, soothing the inflammation, helping ensure that it only responds when it needs to.

Our gut bugs and our immune system are not separate things operating in their own sectioned-off zones. They have a deep, powerful and historical interrelationship. There's even interplay between the composition of your gut bugs and the diet choices you make. That sounds incredible, I know, but your gut bugs can change your mood and these mood changes influence whether you're going to reach for the healthy salad or the super-sweet pastry. Eating different foods also affects your gut bugs in such a way that they alter our body's signaling processes, including how hungry you feel. In these ways and more, these trillions of bacteria that live inside you are taking over your thoughts and influencing your actions every day. It seems profoundly creepy, I know, but remember it works both ways. We can control our gut bugs—and help them work for us—with our food choices.

*"There are actually more immune reactions in your gut, over the course of one day, than the rest of your body in your entire lifetime."*

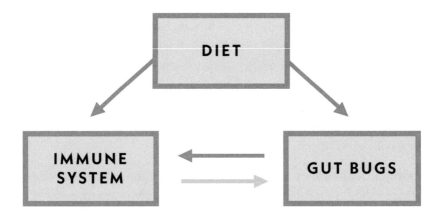

## EATING THE RAINBOW

When you start eating differently, your microbiome will start changing within two to three days. Getting five different vegetables into your diet every single day will accelerate the process of optimizing your microbiome. To enhance the benefits even further, try to make these vegetables as many different colors as you can. This means it's much more likely that you will encourage the growth of more beneficial bacteria as well as getting maximum gut-bug diversity. But that's not the only benefit.

The more colors we eat, the more variety we'll be getting of these incredible compounds that are known as phytonutrients. Many people don't like to eat their vegetables and vegetables themselves don't like to be eaten. Plants generate various compounds, called phytonutrients, to defend themselves against consumption. These defense molecules, when eaten by us, can have a remarkable impact on our health. There are literally thousands of them and we're only just beginning to understand their many benefits. They include many different types such as the polyphenols found in olives (see page 84) as well as the glucosinolates found in cruciferous vegetables such as broccoli, cauliflower, kale, turnips, brussels sprouts and cabbage. We already know that phytonutrients help heart health, fight cancer cells, reduce inflammation and reverse brain aging.

Different colors contain different phytonutrients. Red foods, such as tomatoes, contain lycopene, which some researchers argue reduces the risk of some types of cancer and heart disease. Orange foods, such as carrots, contain beta-carotene, which has a beneficial effect on our immune system and promotes healthy vision. Green vegetables, such as broccoli, contain chlorophyll, which seems to help control hunger. The phytonutrients found in bitter foods such as kale help us feel full. The list goes on. (You even find polyphenols—a particular type of phytonutrient—in delightful products like red wine, coffee and high-quality chocolate—but that's not an excuse to binge!)

# POLYPHENOLS

Polyphenols are a special class of phytonutrients. There are many different types of polyphenol including lignans from flaxseeds, flavonoids found in dark chocolate and red wine, catechins found in tea, and anthocyanins found in broccoli and berries. We're only just beginning to learn about the many different health benefits they confer.

So far we do know that polyphenols have powerful antioxidant effects. Oxidation is a normal process that occurs in the body as a by-product of various physiological functions. If the antioxidant balance is disrupted the result in our bodies can very simplistically be likened to rusting on a car. Polyphenols help to dampen down this rusting process and prevent it from causing damage to our bodies.

Other health benefits may include:

| | |
|---|---|
| Lower inflammation | Improved blood sugar control |
| Slower aging | Improved cardiovascular health |
| Reduced blood pressure | Healthier microbiome |
| Improved brain health | Improved immune function |

## Vegetables

One of the best ways to increase the amount of polyphenols in your diet is by eating brightly colored fiber-rich vegetables. The best sources are spinach, broccoli, red onions, asparagus, red lettuce, shallots, carrots, artichokes and both green and black olives. Polyphenols are typically found in higher concentrations in the skin of fruit and vegetables, so peeling them can remove a large amount.

### Berries

Berries are worth a special mention as they are jam-packed full of polyphenols. I actually highly recommend berries to my patients, in addition to five vegetables per day, because of their high polyphenol content. Their bright colors also make it easier for you to eat the rainbow.

### Other sources

Some of the best sources include dark chocolate, coffee and nuts such as pecans and hazelnuts. The polyphenols found in black and green tea can inhibit the growth of many problematic gut bugs. You can also up your intake with the liberal use of herbs, especially rosemary, thyme and peppermint, and by using copious amounts of extra-virgin olive oil.

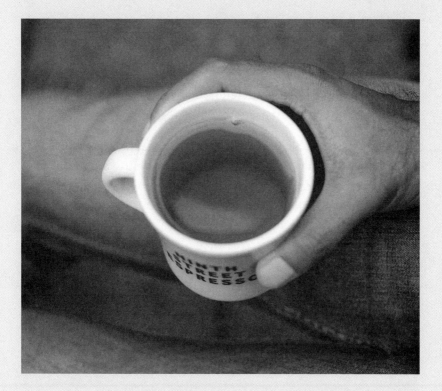

# HOW TO INCREASE YOUR COLORS

Use the rainbow chart on pages 88–89 to help increase the number of colors you consume. My focus with this intervention is primarily to encourage you to eat five different vegetables per day. If you can make them different colors too, so much the better. I have included some non-vegetable items in the chart such as blueberries, nuts, lentils and black rice because of their established health benefits. My hope is that these additional items will help to make your diet more colorful.

Here are some practical tips to help increase your vegetable intake and variety:

- Print out the rainbow chart from drchatterjee.com and put it on your fridge. Check off all the colors you have consumed in one day.

- Involve friends, family or work colleagues to help you stay motivated.

- Get in the habit of snacking on vegetables—carrots with hummus, cucumber with tahini, and celery sticks with almond butter are some tasty options.

- Avocados and olives make a quick and easy snack—although technically fruits, in culinary circles they are treated as vegetables. I consider them to be foods that can be included as part of your new "five a day."

- Leave colorful, appealing vegetables on the kitchen counter or your desk so that you see them regularly: bright orange carrots, slices of red and yellow peppers, green olives.

- Add two vegetables to every meal, including breakfast. If you're having eggs in the morning, try adding spinach and avocado.

- A tip that I use with my children is to serve them their vegetables first. Only when they have eaten them will I dish out the rest of the meal. This works for adults too!

- Roast a whole baking tray of colorful vegetables drizzled with olive oil; eat some with your evening meal and save leftovers in the fridge. They can form the basis of lunch the next day.

# RAINBOW CHART FOR YOU TO COMPLETE

| | GREENS | | REDS |
|---|---|---|---|
| | Artichoke | Cucumber | |
| | Asparagus | Edamame Beans | Red Peppers |
| | Avocado | Green Beans | Beets |
| | Bamboo Shoots | Garden Peas | Red Onions |
| | Green Peppers | Arugula | Red Cabbage |
| | Bok Choy | Spinach | Radish |
| | ~~Broccoli~~ | ~~Lettuce~~ | ~~Rhubarb~~ |
| | Brussels Sprouts | Swiss Chard | Tomato |
| | Cabbage | Kale | Radicchio |
| | Celery | Okra | |

MONDAY

TUESDAY

WEDNESDAY

THURSDAY

FRIDAY

SATURDAY

SUNDAY

| ORANGES | YELLOWS | PURPLES | WHITES |
|---|---|---|---|
| | | Olives | Chickpeas |
| | | Purple Carrots | Cauliflower |
| | | Purple Sweet | Mushrooms |
| Carrots | Corn | Potatoes | Shallots |
| Orange Peppers | Yellow Peppers | Kale | Seeds |
| Pumpkin | Ginger Root | Purple Potatoes | Onions |
| Butternut Squash | Summer Squash | Blueberries | Garlic |
| Sweet Potato | Lemons | Red Cabbage | Turnips |
| Turmeric Root | | Black Rice | Fennel |
| | | Eggplant | Nuts |
| | | | Lentils |
| | | | Parsnips |

# 3. INTRODUCE DAILY MICRO-FASTS

*Get into the habit of eating all of your food*

*within a twelve-hour time window.*

Humans evolved during periods of regular feast and famine. Our bodies are designed for going without food for certain periods of time. But the modern environment, in which we're surrounded by temptations to eat—be they social pressures, via advertising or the simple fact we have that delicious half-eaten tub of ice cream sitting in our freezer—means we tend to inundate our systems.

As soon as you start to give your body a break from all the gorging, incredible things start to happen. An extraordinary health-promoting cascade effect is triggered. After six to eight hours, the liver will have used up its internal fuel stores, in the form of glycogen, and soon after this the body will start to burn its own fat. Once we get to about twelve hours, a process called autophagy will have well and truly kicked in.

Autophagy is another hot area of new research that I wasn't taught about in medical school. Much of what we know about it is thanks to the Japanese biologist Yoshinori Ohsumi, who won the Nobel Prize in Medicine for his work into its mechanisms. Imagine that you never spent time cleaning up your house. You'd leave dirty plates hanging around for weeks, stinky clothes on the floor, kids' toys everywhere, laundry baskets overflowing, the sinks machine-gunned with toothpaste splats. This is basically what happens in the body, every day, as a by-product of it going about its daily functions. The scientific term for this is "oxidative damage." It's actually a little bit like the rust that builds up on cars. This build-up is an inevitable consequence of function—and it's all fine as long as we give our body a chance to clean up. This is what autophagy does. Think of it as your built-in Cinderella. It's your body sorting out its mess and busying itself with cellular repair, immune system repair and a host of other essential maintenance projects. Eating all your food in a restricted time window—for example, within twelve hours—allows your body to enhance its own natural house-cleaning.

Being such a new area of science, there's still limited data on human studies into exactly how and why time-restricted feeding (TRF) assists our repair processes. However, one likely mechanism that's been proposed is that when we don't eat for several hours, the liver stops secreting glucose into the bloodstream and instead uses it to repair cell damage. The liver is simultaneously stimulated to release enzymes that break down stored fat and cholesterol. Therefore, during our fasting period, the liver is helping to repair our bodies and burn off fat!

And these are by no means the only benefits of restricting our hours of eating. An incredible American neurologist, Dr. Dale Bredesen, has actually managed to reverse memory loss in early-Alzheimer's patients by taking a multipronged approach that has, as an essential component, regular twelve-hour fasts. Yet more compelling research is coming out of the lab of Dr. Satchidananda Panda, a biologist at the Salk Institute for Biological Studies in San Diego. Dr. Panda is a passionate promoter of the idea that restricting the timing of our food intake may be an extremely effective public health stratagem. He argues that simply trying to eliminate unhealthy foods and restrict calories hasn't really proved successful—so perhaps a limited eating window might work better.

If all that wasn't enough, early studies are showing that when animals are given exactly the same diets over varying time periods, the metabolic effects on their body are significantly different—they put on less fat and have larger muscle mass when they are fed over a shorter period. This is hugely exciting. Human trials are under way.

So far the reported benefits are:

| | |
|---|---|
| **Lower levels of inflammation** | **Enhanced detoxification— TRF improves the elimination of waste products** |
| **Improved blood sugar control** | |
| **Improved mitochondrial function (see box opposite)** | **Increased production of Akkermansia muciniphila (see page 78)** |
| **Improved immune function** | **Improved appetite signaling** |

It is possible to enhance these benefits by shortening our eating window even further, but I recommend twelve hours because fasting for longer can be problematic for some. Most patients I see are chronically overstressed. They need more rest-and-recuperation time, not more time under stress. Although perhaps not truly optimal, twelve hours is both manageable and long enough for most of us to see real benefits.

# MITOCHONDRIA

Mitochondria are the energy factories of your body. Every cell contains hundreds of thousands of them. They convert fuel, in the form of oxygen and food, into energy. If we want to reach optimal health, we should try to enhance mitochondrial function in any way we can.

Most mitochondria are found in highly active organs such as the brain and the heart and in muscle tissue. Mitochondrial function is central to almost every single physiological process in the body.

Poor mitochondrial function can result in:

- Low energy level
- Brain fog
- Pain
- Poor memory
- Premature aging

As mitochondria produce energy, reactive oxygen species (ROS) are formed. These cause oxidation, which is a bit like rusting on a car. In order to mop these potentially harmful reactive oxygen species up, our bodies need to produce sufficient antioxidants from the fruit and vegetables in our diet. Small amounts of these ROS are helpful, but too many causes problems.

When mitochondria don't function optimally, the increase in ROS is known as increased oxidative stress.

In the short or medium term, this can contribute to the symptoms listed above such as fatigue and poor memory. Over the long term, this leads to chronic inflammation which can be a significant driver of many different diseases in the body including obesity, type 2 diabetes and stroke.

Eating an anti-inflammatory whole-food diet (see "Unprocess Your Diet" on page 104) helps provide mitochondria with the correct fuel and necessary repair materials. In addition, the mitochondrial walls are made up of fat, so having healthy sources of natural fat in your diet such as avocados, olive oil and oily fish is important. Mitochondria also need the right fuel, which can be obtained from eating an anti-inflammatory whole-food diet.

Which twelve hours should you choose? Recently I experimented by not eating after 7 p.m. I found it surprisingly easy. As it turned out, eating later was just habit, just as feeling hungry later was a habit, mostly based upon the readily available access to food in my house. When I stopped eating during the evenings I felt more energetic, had better sleep and was just generally a little lighter in myself. I came to think of that evening craving for food as having a kind of "itchy mouth." That's become the way we talk about it in my house now. Am I really hungry? Or do I just have an itchy mouth?

## WORKING WITH YOUR CIRCADIAN RHYTHM

Although the science in this area is still in its infancy, human studies are already hinting that scheduling an earlier evening meal, or skipping it completely, may be more beneficial than not having breakfast. This appears to be because certain bodily functions shut down and don't function optimally in the evening. Intuitively, this makes a lot of sense, but in the scientific world this is actually quite surprising. Isn't a body like a machine? As in, it either works or it doesn't? Why should one bit of it work better at a certain time of day?

I find it incredibly exciting that much of our biological machinery actually has its own daily cycle, not dissimilar to the one that makes us feel sleepy or alert at different points of the day. Even if we're not deeply familiar with the science of the "circadian rhythm"—how the body floods with melatonin to make us drowsy and cortisol to wake us up—we'll certainly be aware of its effects. It's now becoming clear that our bodies work on any number of these kinds of routine cycles.

Last year I was on my way to a conference in San Diego and, on the plane from Manchester to Heathrow, I happened to find myself sitting next to Andrew Louden, a professor of animal biology from the University of Manchester. We started chatting and before I knew it, we'd landed. We both had some time to wait before our next flight so continued the conversation over coffee. As I sipped at my short black Americano, I mentioned I was traveling to a conference on sleep cycles and I started talking to him about body clocks. "Well, yes, I actually study body clocks," he chuckled. "And it's not all about sleep, you know. Did you know that if you take a bunch of human liver cells and put them in a test tube, they start operating by daily rhythms?"

I found this extraordinary. Andrew told me that all of our bodily functions are determined by a circadian rhythm. This made me wonder if one potentially major failing of many health and nutrition studies might be that they haven't accounted for this. When I looked into it, I found some fascinating recent research to suggest that certain pharmaceutical drugs could work better at different times of the day. Certain genes are also more or less active at various points. Even the composition of our gut microbiome changes with the hours. Interestingly enough, traditional Chinese medicine has been making this kind of observation for thousands of years. They've long believed that various organs have increased function at certain times of the day.

# SIX TIPS TO HELP YOU MICRO-FAST

1. Choose a twelve-hour period that suits your lifestyle. Note that your twelve-hour eating window is from the beginning of your first meal to the end of your last meal.

2. Your body likes rhythm, so try and keep to the same times every day, even on the weekends. Occasionally you may need to change your eating window—this is absolutely fine.

3. Outside your eating window, stick to water, herbal tea or black tea and coffee. Be careful with caffeine so you don't adversely affect your sleep (see page 205).

4. Try to involve other members of your household, or even work colleagues. This will help to keep you motivated and increase your chances of success.

5. Don't be disheartened if you miss a day, or even two. It really doesn't matter. When you feel ready, try again and see how you get on.

6. When you are feeling comfortable with twelve hours, you may choose to experiment with shorter eating windows on different days. If you do this, pay attention to how the change makes you feel and adjust accordingly.

All this explains why it's a good idea to start your time-restricted feeding window earlier. Hunter-gatherers tended to do their "work" either in the morning or at twilight. Have our bodies kept this ancient programming and could this be one of the reasons that gene activity, for example, peaks at these times? I don't think we know the exact answer to this question yet, but it seems logical. If you ask me, we're not meant to be eating just before we're about to go to bed. We've evolved to eat in the light. Indeed, researchers in Scandinavia found that, in some people, when the body is preparing to sleep, and we're feeling tired, the pancreas stops making insulin. You can't override that. Today, we're eating out of sync with our natural rhythms. Time-restricted feeding helps us readjust and give the body what it's expecting at the time it's expecting it. This helps it make the most efficient use of the fuel we swallow.

# 4. DRINK MORE WATER

*Aim to drink eight small glasses*
*(approximately 1.2 liters) of water per day.*

Do you feel tired? Or regularly experience low-grade and long-lasting headaches? Often when worried patients come in complaining of symptoms such as these, it turns out that many of them are simply not drinking enough water.

Now the idea we should be drinking eight glasses of water a day has been around for many years but, interestingly enough, there's not actually that much science to support it. That doesn't mean I'm not going to recommend it, however. What should I do as a practicing doctor? Wait for the evidence to come from academia that frankly may never arrive? Or should I make a sensible recommendation that I've seen help thousands of patients? I choose to help patients now.

This is the big difference between researchers and clinicians. Researchers assess evidence but it can be a long time before such evidence gets translated into mainstream clinical practice—some say about thirty years! In addition, some concepts never get properly examined, sometimes because they're hard to study, but often because there's simply no financial imperative to do so. I always remember my chat with the inspiring Olympic strength coach Charles Poliquin: "If you wait for the evidence, you may miss three Olympic cycles," he told me. That idea has resonated with me ever since.

About 60 percent of the body is made up of water and we can only last a few days without it. Water helps us digest food and process substances such as alcohol. Losing just 2 percent of body weight in fluid can actually reduce our physical and mental performance by up to 25 percent. I've seen a host of different ailments clear up when people start drinking more water, including headaches, low energy levels, dry skin and stomachache. It can even be helpful for constipation. If you're feeling tired and sluggish in the afternoon, it could simply be that you are slightly dehydrated. I've experienced this myself on many occasions (not least while writing this book).

## DON'T DRINK YOUR CALORIES

As someone who abides by the Hippocratic oath, one of my first criteria with any recommendation I make is, how much harm can it do? The only potential downside to this one is maybe a couple more trips to the bathroom. But that's it, and even that helps you increase your daily activity level, which I'd chalk up as a benefit. In addition, drinking more water will hopefully mean you start drinking less of the sweetened stuff, such as juices and soft drinks. Fluid bypasses normal satiety mechanisms in the body and allows us to consume a lot more energy and calories than would be possible if we were eating. Think about oranges as an example. A glass of orange juice could easily have six or seven oranges in it. It's perfectly possible to drink a whole glass in one go whereas it's very difficult to eat six or seven oranges at a sitting. Whole oranges also contain fiber that slows the release of sugar into the body. Juicing removes that beneficial fiber.

And don't think you can necessarily get around this by sticking to diet drinks. A correlation has been found between zero-calorie soft drinks and disorders such as diabetes. While the science isn't able to say definitively that drinking these products causes these problems, it certainly remains a distinct possibility. There are several plausible mechanisms we know of that could explain how this might happen. One theory has it that diet drinks contain chemicals that can have an

## HEALTH BENEFITS YOU MAY EXPERIENCE FROM DRINKING MORE WATER

Fewer headaches

Increased energy levels

Better bowel function

Clearer skin

Fewer stomachaches

Longer periods of concentration

Reduced cravings for sugar

adverse impact on the gut microbiome. As we've already learned, our microbiome health is critical for good health. While we're waiting for the science to catch up, I'd advocate not taking the risk, and cutting out diet drinks too.

A patient of mine named Annabelle had been suffering from headaches for years and had tried many different medications unsuccessfully. These headaches didn't really follow any pattern and she was getting extremely frustrated by them. When I first met her, I got the sense that she wasn't drinking enough water. I asked her to aim for eight small glasses per day. In less than a week, her headaches completely vanished. An added bonus was that she had more energy as well.

Again, I must stress that I'm aware of no study that points to eight glasses as being optimal. It's simply impossible for me to state with accuracy what your individual requirements are. It depends on so many variables, including the kind of job you have, the physical size of your body and even the climate in which you live. But in my years of clinical experience I've found that eight small glasses seems to be about right for most people, most of the time. A simple rule of thumb is to look at your urine. You're aiming for a color that is light yellow to clear.

Many people—my father-in-law included—find it extremely difficult to get anywhere near eight glasses of water per day. For people like him, I've come up with some simple strategies. First thing in the morning drink two glasses. If you'd prefer some flavor in it, try squeezing some lemon in there. Before you've even started filling up with breakfast, you're already two glasses down. Another helpful strategy is to add in a glass of water thirty minutes before each meal.

# TIPS TO HELP YOU INCREASE
# YOUR WATER INTAKE

HAVE TWO GLASSES OF WATER WHEN YOU
WAKE UP EACH MORNING ✓

IF YOU'RE HUNGRY MID-MORNING OR
MID-AFTERNOON, TRY HAVING A GLASS OF
WATER INSTEAD OF A SNACK ✓

ONCE EVERY HOUR, GET UP FROM YOUR DESK
AND GO TO THE WATER COOLER ✓

DRINK A GLASS OF WATER THIRTY MINUTES
BEFORE EACH MEAL ✓

SET AN ALARM THREE TIMES PER DAY
TO REMIND YOU TO HAVE A DRINK ✓

TRY ADDING LEMON OR ORANGE SLICES
FOR FLAVOR ✓

BUY A 20-OUNCE WATER BOTTLE. WE'RE AIMING
FOR 1.2 LITERS PER DAY, SO TRY TO HAVE
FINISHED ONE BY LUNCH AND ONE BY DINNER ✓

There is some evidence suggesting that drinking water thirty minutes before meals may reduce the amount of calories you consume. Then, if you start feeling hunger pangs in the middle of the morning or mid-afternoon, try having a couple of glasses of water instead between meals.

If you implement some of the above strategies, you should be well on your way in no time.

# 5. UNPROCESS YOUR DIET

*Try to avoid food products that contain more than five ingredients.*

There's no need to count calories, portion size, fats, carbs, Weight Watchers points or anything even remotely like that. Life is complicated enough as it is. Instead, simply focus on avoiding highly processed foods. It's a pretty safe bet that any food product that contains more than five ingredients is highly processed. By avoiding these foods you will, by default, be not only improving your health but also side-stepping all the endless confusion that exists about diet. All you need to do is remember the number five.

Our ideas about food have become too reductionist. We've been beguiled by powerful diet cults that are desperate to convert us to their passionate belief that they have found the One True Diet. Everyone—including me—has been swept up in these debates and harbors their own personal biases about what's good and bad. For years we were told that the answer lay in counting calories, despite the fact that a healthy avocado contains more than double the calories of a can of Coke. Do they both have the same effect on the body? Of course not. (And we know which has more than five ingredients!)

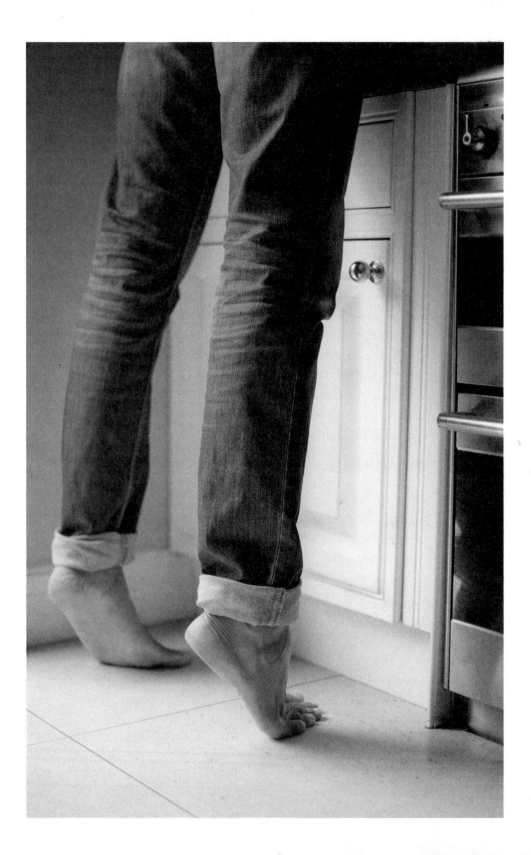

# 3. BEGIN REGULAR HIGH-INTENSITY INTERVAL TRAINING

*Find a form of HIIT that works for you and do two ten- to fifteen-minute sessions each week.*

What if I told you it was possible to exercise less and achieve more? Would you believe me? Or would you think I was hawking some too-good-to-be true "wellness" scheme and was about to ask you to buy an $800 gadget and sign some byzantine contract? The amazing fact of the matter is, a lot of modern science is telling us exactly that. High-intensity interval training—often shortened to HIIT—is a very specific form of training that's been shown to have some fantastic health benefits. In simple terms, it refers to exercising hard, but in short bursts.

Health benefits include:

| | |
|---|---|
| Slowing the aging process | Losing dangerous, internal visceral fat (see page 145) |
| Increasing the growth of brain cells | Increasing mitochondrial numbers and function |
| Improving insulin sensitivity, which helps prevent type 2 diabetes | Losing weight |

Back in my early days as a GP, I used to stop at the gym on the way to work. I needed to be at my desk by 7:30 a.m. to start going through paperwork, blood results and all the other important but time-consuming items that pile up on a doctor's desk before they even start seeing patients. I'd leave my house at 6:20 to ensure I'd be at the gym when it opened at 6:30. It would take me about five minutes to check in, change and get to the equipment. From 6:35 until 6:55 I'd work out, jumping from side to side, sprinting on the squash court, lunging up and down the gym and maybe finishing off with some weights. By 7:10 I was back in my work clothes, freshly shaved and showered. I'd arrive at my office at about 7:25 and was ready to go with my computer all set up at 7:30.

One of my colleagues at the office said to me, "What's the point of just going for twenty minutes? You may as well not bother." She was a GP and this was her strong belief. In fact, she was someone who used to battle with her weight and always found the gym a struggle. She'd only go when she had a full hour to dedicate to it, otherwise she felt she was wasting her time. This was a big mistake. And yet I see it being made every day by friends, colleagues and patients. The fact is, you do not need to dedicate all that much time to working out.

Whether you're spending too much time in the gym or not enough, HIIT could be the answer. The difference between HIIT and a traditional exercise session is that, rather than going non-stop for an extended period of time, your workout is sectioned off into lots of smaller sessions, with "intervals" of rest in between them. And these sessions must be intense. By that I mean they should be intense for you. I want you to be pushing yourself. You should go all out, sweat running, heart pumping. By the end, you should be out of breath and unable to hold a conversation for a good thirty seconds. This sounds tough, but it's important to remember that you only have to do this for a short period of time. You'll feel recovered again pretty quickly.

The evidence that the body responds better to this form of training is powerful and growing. One recent study found that an eleven-minute HIIT workout gives as much benefit as one hour of continuous activity. Another, by one of the world's leading researchers into HIIT, Martin Gibala, showed that one minute of intense working out, pushing yourself as hard as you possibly can in three twenty-second bursts of intense cycling spread out over ten minutes, showed equivalent improvement to forty-five minutes of moderate-intensity cycling. Think about these numbers for a moment. They're truly incredible. It's surely little wonder the famous journalist A. A. Gill once wondered if HIIT could be "the most time saving invention since the microwave."

Just as impressive are the positive threshold effects that HIIT has on our massively connected bodies. HIIT improves our insulin sensitivity much more than ordinary forms of exercise, making us less likely to contract type 2 diabetes. It improves our mitochondrial function, which enables all bodily processes to work better. It reduces inflammation. It makes our blood vessels work more efficiently. It increases cardiorespiratory fitness. It's really good for weight loss. The very latest research on HIIT is even hinting that it might slow the aging process. Researchers from the Mayo Clinic published a study in March 2017 which found that HIIT may reverse aging at the cellular level.

## VISCERAL FAT

There are lots of different types of fat in the human body that are classified not only by their actual structure but also by where they're found. One particularly dangerous kind is called "visceral fat." People can look as if they don't have a weight problem, but when you put them in a scanner, you discover that they have layers of internal fat covering their organs. This is visceral fat. People sometimes refer to sufferers of the condition as TOFI—"thin on the outside, fat on the inside." Just because you look thin, it doesn't necessarily follow that you are thin. What's more, visceral fat is more dangerous than what we call "subcutaneous" fat, which is the stuff that lies just beneath the skin. It puts you at increased risk of heart attacks and stroke. And guess what? HIIT is especially good at getting rid of visceral fat.

## BUILDING BRAIN HEALTH

What about brain health? We know all kinds of exercise are helpful for our cognition, but one 2015 study found that HIIT helps increase something called "brain-derived neurotrophic factor," or BDNF. BDNF is a supportive molecule for the brain. Think of it like high-octane fuel. It helps prevent terrible brain disorders such as dementia. It grows new nerve cells. Another study showed that just twenty minutes of aerobic exercise a day can increase BDNF as well as the growth of cells in the hippocampus, which is the part of your brain responsible for memory. There's no pharmaceutical drug that can increase BDNF and, if there were, everyone on earth would want it. And yet movement can do this—especially HIIT.

But which particular form of exercise increases BDNF the most? This—at least at the moment—is very hard to say. However, one exciting study showed that following intense, rather than low-intensity, exercise, people not only learned vocabulary 20 percent faster but also had bigger spikes in their BDNF levels. Could there be an additional benefit for HIIT? I think so.

## CHOOSING THE WORKOUT THAT WORKS FOR YOU

There are a lot of different versions of HIIT, but I like to think of it as any form of exercise in which there's a sudden change in activity that forces your body to adapt. It must be a period of high-intensity movement followed by a period of low-intensity movement.

And it must be "intense" as perceived by you. My aim with this book is to help you simplify health. This is why I don't want you measuring your pulse or counting your breathing rate. As long as you perceive it as very hard, it works for me. For example, if you like going to the gym, you can jump on a treadmill and do forty seconds at perhaps 7.5 miles per hour (or whatever pace feels very hard to you), then, for one minute and twenty seconds, go at 2.5 miles per hour, which will be much easier. That sharp change forces your body to adapt physiologically. Doing it in bursts gives you much more benefit for your buck. Repeat this three to five times.

But it doesn't have to be that hard. It all depends upon your current fitness levels. It doesn't even have to be in a gym. One of my most popular workouts (featured in the first series of my BBC show, *Doctor in the House*) is one of the simplest. Many of my patients love it for the ease with which it fits into their everyday life. It works like this. Walk out of your front door and go to the end of your road.

From there, walk as fast as you can for one minute. When that minute's over, look to see which house number you've arrived at, then walk at a normal pace back to the start. Now you repeat the same sequence, but this time you want to see if you can beat yourself and get to a house further down the road. This may sound relatively easy, but by the time you have done this three times, you will be really feeling it. Try and do this five times altogether. It will only take you ten or fifteen minutes maximum, you don't need a gym membership or fancy clothes and the benefits are profound.

Don't want to go outside on a rainy October day? Fine. How about doing ten burpees, ten jumping jacks and ten side lunges sequentially in your living room for forty seconds? Then spend the next eighty seconds walking around slowly and then repeat five times. Alternatively, try a combination of fast alternating leg lunges, push-ups and kettlebell swings. If none of these appeal, make up your own. There are infinite possibilities!

# 4. MOVEMENT SNACKING

*Make a habit of doing three or four "movement snacks"*
*five days a week.*

One of my favorite quotes is from George Bernard Shaw, who said, "We don't stop playing because we grow old; we grow old because we stop playing." This is all too true and I've no doubt that one of the reasons we find our health and energy levels deteriorating (and thus put on weight) as we grow older is that we're no longer running around having fun—playing tag, kicking a ball around, skipping on the playground. I'd love it if it became the norm among us grown-up children that we rediscovered this part of our nature, which becomes repressed as all the responsibilities of adulthood pile in and weigh us down. Imagine if, in offices up and down the country, everyone did a two-minute workout together before they went out for lunch! Some quick lunges, dips, air squats or side lunges would be amazing for company team-building and morale and even better for the nation's health.

This intervention is focused on fun and play. One of the reasons people who engage in sport tend to stick with their regimens so well is because they're doing it for pleasure. I've recently rediscovered the joy I find in playing squash. I get to unwind, engage my competitive side and, by default, I work up a sweat and improve my health. Not only that, I also feel fantastic afterward. I play with one of my elementary school buddies and it's not unusual for us to just spend the first ten minutes laughing and ribbing each other. Those forty-five minutes are golden for me. I simply cannot wait for my weekly game.

# PLAYING TOGETHER

Doing our movement snacks in company really helps, whether it's with your partner, your friends or your fellow workers. And it doesn't have to be something long and intense like a game of squash. What I'm really talking about here is little bite-sized snacks of movement. Grab a jump rope, do a load of jumping jacks or race your colleagues around the office. When I am at home, I will dive onto the floor (or go in the garden) and mimic various animal moves with the kids: an ape, a bear, a frog or a crab. Fun as well as energizing—it leaves us all breathless. We change it up every day but it could be squats, primal tag (see below), step-ups on the stairs . . . Sometimes we just put some music on and start singing and dancing. It drives my wife crazy but we have a complete laugh. By the time we start eating dinner, we're often a little out of breath. The fantastic thing about doing these movement snacks before eating is that they actually change the way your body deals with your meal. Several studies have shown that when you do some exercise immediately before food, your blood sugar rises less after you've eaten.

One of my favorite games was introduced to me by a friend called Darryl Edwards, creator of the Primal Play Method. He calls it Primal Play Tag. You need two people and the aim is simply to try to touch your opponent between the knee and the hip. So you're both simultaneously trying to avoid and trying to tag. This is three-dimensional movement. You can do it pretty much anywhere, and it's so much fun that you just don't feel like you're exercising.

# THE KITCHEN GYM

For me, the kitchen has always been a fantastic place to indulge in a quick movement snack. I remember as a teenager, I'd use the two minutes it took for my food to warm up in the microwave to hit the deck and bang out some push-ups. Nowadays, I do twenty squats with my kids in the time it takes for spinach to steam. You could take two bottles of olive oil and lift them up over your head and to the sides, hop on each leg for thirty seconds or even simply jump from side to side. The point is to get your heart pumping three or four times a day—but it has to be fun!

# THE OFFICE WORKOUT

I'd love it to become the norm in offices to have a little play-based movement snack at the start of lunch every day. You could do a combination of the movements mentioned below or devise your own. How about starting every lunch break with the following? Dare as many of your colleagues as you can to join in:

1. Five triceps dips on your desk (see triceps dips on page 138)

2. Five jumping jacks

3. Five hand clap lunges on each leg—Stand opposite a partner and do a lunge toward each other. As you do, use your left hand to do a high five with their left hand.

4. Five side lunges on each leg—Step to the left. Keep your body facing forward and your right foot planted on the floor, while bending your left knee.

5. Five desk push-ups (see push-ups on page 138)

This is meant to be fun. No judgment. No competition. Just a way of engaging everyone to be active. The great thing about doing this as a group is that it is much more likely to become permanent. Some days you won't feel like doing it but your colleagues will. Hopefully, that will be the motivation to do this every day at work! It's easy to fall into the trap of thinking that small bursts of movement like these won't have much effect, but it's these little things you do every day that translate into the big health outcomes. The truth is, good health isn't meant to be that hard, nor is it meant to be boring.

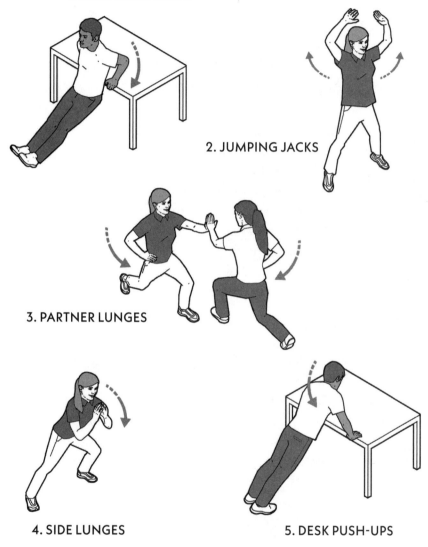

1. DESK TRICEPS DIPS

2. JUMPING JACKS

3. PARTNER LUNGES

4. SIDE LUNGES

5. DESK PUSH-UPS

# 5. WAKE UP YOUR SLEEPY GLUTES

*Do at least one glute movement every day,*

*and the whole series four times per week.*

Would you build your house on shaky foundations? Would you teach your kids to construct their Lego creations on a sloping floor? Would you stack Jenga blocks on jelly? Well, that's the sort of thing I see many people doing these days with their bodies. Because of modern life, our basic movement mechanics simply aren't working anymore. We spend our days in bent-over postures and our bodies adapt. We mold into the shapes in which we spend most of our waking time. We're hunched over, our shoulders slumped, our feet dragging. We're a generation who has sleepy glute muscles and flat butts.

The reason our glutes have gone to sleep is because of our modern living environment. Our lifestyles have done this to us. The way we live modern life is literally a pain in the ass. And this matters. We usually think of our bottoms as something to sit on, but they're actually one of the most important muscles in the body. They're a "keystone" muscle and, if they're off, there can be ripple effects for many other muscles. A lot of back pain is actually caused by having sleepy backsides. Glutes—our buttock muscles—not only help hold our skeletons up, they play a critical role in the functioning of our biomechanics. It's not by accident that men and women tend to, consciously or unconsciously, judge the quality of a potential mate partly on the shape of their butt. And our glutes do not exist in isolation. In our massively connected bodies, they're linked to a whole chain of muscles from our shoulders all the way down to our feet, and if they're not firing appropriately, that puts stress on other parts of the body.

I know firsthand how important these muscles are. When I was twenty-three I was a final-year medical student at Edinburgh University. I was moving into a new apartment for the year with my friends Steve and Mary. I was helping Mary move boxes up six flights of stairs with the most appalling posture you've ever seen. After about thirty minutes, I lifted a new set of boxes and boom! Sharp pain in my lower right back. I dropped all the boxes and fell to the ground in agony. My back had gone. Up until that point, I'd never given my back any thought. Like most of us, I abused it every day, as I'd never been given any reason not to. This led to ten years of chronic back pain which impacted all aspects of my life. I had to take time off work, carefully plan travel and give up all the sports that I loved.

I spent hours, not to mention lots of money, seeking a solution. Everyone told me that, because of my height (I'm six foot six), back pain was inevitable. I simply refused to accept this and tried what felt like every therapy known to man. Most of them would give me short-term relief but within weeks the pain would come back. My desire to learn more led to me signing up to learn about movement mechanics with one of the subject's most revolutionary thinkers, Gary Ward. Gary is an incredibly important figure in the world of body mechanics and human movement. He's flipping all the old rules on their head and having great success in helping people. The brilliance of Gary's philosophy is that he's managed to simplify the huge complexity of the body's mechanics. Using his perspective, we can now work with the idea that the body's movements can be separated and worked with in just two primary chains.

## FLEXOR CHAIN MUSCLES

The first one is the flexor chain. When we're curling our biceps or bringing our knees up to our chests, we're flexing. In our modern environment we tend to overuse our flexor chain. We're flexing our spines from the minute we get up to the minute we go to bed. We gawp at our smartphones with a flexed neck. A human head weighs between nine and eleven pounds, which is a big load to put on our neck joints each time we do this. We sit down to eat breakfast, sit down to get to work, hunch over a desk all day and then come home to sit on a sofa. This takes its toll. One of the main problems with sitting so much is that we're not giving our bodies the chance to experience the opposite posture. Things are so bad for many of us that we actually remain in this hunched, flexed state even when we do stand up! Clues that we are overusing our flexor chain include:

- Flat feet
- Knock knees
- Rounded upper back
- Forward head posture
- Sleepy glutes

## EXTENSOR CHAIN MUSCLES

The opposite of the flexor chain is the extensor chain. We're using our extensor chain when our hips or spines are extended and upright. The muscles of extension enable us to stand up tall with our eyes on the horizon—the very opposite, in fact, of bad posture. The role of the extensor chain is to activate and pull us out of our flexed states. The key to achieving balance in our posture is to have full access to them both, so that the brain can choose what is optimal for the body's environment.

When the body's flexor and extensor chains are working together in balance, you see the classic "book on head" posture:

- Standing up tall

- Long neck

- Head back

- Shoulders back and down

- Ribcage raised and elevated

- Glutes firing, active and switched on

Consciously trying to make these changes is not usually a successful long-term strategy. I spent years trying to implement the old commandment of pulling the shoulders back and standing up straight but it didn't work because I was not re-educating my brain. Gary's approach is aimed at moving the body to wake these extensor chain muscles up, switch your glutes on and make you stand up tall without even having to think about it.

Because we spend so much of our modern lives hunched over, we've lost the ability to extend and be upright. We've got this almost fetal-like flexed posture from sitting in chairs and looking at screens and phones all day. A lot of the corrective work that people find themselves having to undergo involves restoring their powers of extension. When we fail to access our own extensor chain, one of the major muscle groups that deactivates and goes to sleep is the glutes.

# EXTEND, EXTEND, EXTEND

This has been my mantra for the past few years and I hope it will become yours as well! We need to re-teach our body to extend. People struggle to extend their hips, people struggle to extend their spines. Of course, sitting less is extremely helpful but it doesn't automatically allow our bodies to experience extension. Most of us will need help in order to access our body's powers of extension in full.

When people are working on their bodies today, they tend to focus too much on the "mirror muscles," which are the ones you can see in the mirror and so, naturally, the ones they prefer to work on. They get caught up in exercises that make the mirror muscles look good, such as bench presses, biceps curls and sit-ups. All these exercises ask the body to flex. We need far more focus on the muscles we can't see in the mirror, such as the ones on our back that extend the body and make it stand up straight.

As a teenager, a classic tall, skinny Indian kid, I remember being in the changing room at school and I could see my ribs. That made me extremely self-conscious. Meanwhile, I was being exposed to pictures of buff men in all the fitness magazines. I started doing chest presses and sit-ups every day. I kept this up for about two years and, yes, I put on muscle. But I also inadvertently changed all of my body movement mechanics. Was it worth it? Absolutely not. I had to spend years in pain and then years of corrective exercising to undo the damage I'd caused. My mistake was being motivated purely by vanity and focusing on the mirror muscles. I see this whenever I'm in a gym—bodybuilders with overflexed and hunched shoulders, flat feet and rounded spines clearly walking around with poor posture and limited mobility.

I've always prided myself on being particularly open-minded as a doctor and I'm always enthusiastic about learning new things from different healthcare professionals. I was actually the first medical doctor to study with Gary, and what blew my mind about him was the fact that he saw the body in exactly the same way that I saw health. He was motivated by a desire to understand the root cause of problems, rather than simply suppress bodily symptoms. When I came to him with my back problem he very quickly identified that my right foot was "stuck" in pronation. In other words, my foot arch had effectively collapsed and my foot was flat and so unable to access its opposite posture. Podiatrists had told me about my flat foot before but simply prescribed orthotic insoles, which hadn't worked.

Gary had a different solution. He told me he needed to get my right foot working again, insisting that was the key to my back problems. But, you might be thinking, what has this got to do with glutes? Well, in our massively connected bodies, there's actually a strong link between our foot muscles and our glute muscles. If one of our feet isn't working properly, this can directly affect our glutes, and vice versa. It turned out that my right glute muscle wasn't switching on and this meant my back was always going to struggle. My back was taking the strain instead of my sleepy backside.

Under Gary's guidance, it soon became clear why none of those, from physical therapists to massage therapists, who'd been manipulating my back over the years had solved the problem. They'd only ever been offering a temporary Band-Aid fix. To completely heal my back, Gary had to teach me to reprogram these damaging patterns and re-educate my body. I had to get my feet working correctly again. This, in turn, would reawaken my glute muscles. Incredibly, with just five minutes of exercise per day, over the course of less than a week, my long-standing back problems vanished. My exercises were based largely on the four I have detailed at the end of this section (see page 160). It was the nearest thing to a miracle I've ever witnessed. Now, a few years on, I have a natural right-foot arch, my right glute is firing appropriately and my back pain has never resurfaced.

*Thanks to Gary, my body has returned to its natural state. I'm now back to playing squash and skiing down mogul runs with no concerns at all. This has been completely life-changing for me. Day to day, I'm able to move my body more freely, re-engage with activities that I love but had to previously shun. This has had tremendous ripple effects. I'm happier and fitter, and I have more energy and an improved sense of well-being. I'm living a life that was completely unimaginable to me only six years ago.*

It was in Gary's brilliant book *What the Foot?* and in his training courses that I first learned about the importance of glutes, and how we must reawaken them in order to combat the effects of our flexed, hunched-over lifestyles. The glutes are extensor chain muscles. They aid the extension of the hip, which is the motion we make when standing up or coming out of a squat (as opposed to the flexion we make when bending at the hip to sit down). Hip extension and glute contraction should happen together. But in our super-flexed world, we're missing the ability to extend our hips properly. I want you to learn how to move your whole body to access hip extension using the following four exercises. I believe that these exercises will give your body the opportunity to awaken your glutes forevermore.

Some of you might have been through the rigmarole of extending your hips after many a physical therapy session and you might even have come to the conclusion that it doesn't work. If so, I suspect, your discomforts have continued. But this is where Gary's unique philosophy kicks in. He believes that we've become flexed to such an extent that when we even try to extend, using the traditional exercises, we slip into bad habits. Our bodies have simply forgotten how to move as they should. Whenever we stand up, we're supposed to be using our glutes. Most of us don't. Our brains bypass the glutes, using other muscles. In order to retrain the brain, Gary has created a series of exercises that invite it to fire the right muscles. The important thing to know is that we can't simply consciously "decide" to use our glutes and therefore extend properly. Our brains make these decisions for us, unconsciously. Therefore, we need exercises that remind the brain how to trigger the correct muscles. And this is exactly what Gary has designed.

Here's just one example. By bending the hip fully, we create a situation in which the only movement left available is one of proper extension. When we lie on our front and lift one of our legs, we should be doing it using our glute. But when instructed to do this, the brain has many options. Because our glutes are switched off, it tends to choose easier ones. Gary's movements make it so the brain has no option but to lift the leg in the proper way, using the glute.

Gary and I have come up with four movements that are designed to get your feet moving, your hips extending and your glutes firing. They'll help retrain your brain to operate your body in accordance with the way it was designed. They can be carried out individually or as part of a group.

**Note: All movements should be made either barefoot or with socks on.**

# MOVEMENT ONE: FLEX ON A STEP

This can be any exercise step like a standard aerobics step, a baby step stool or even your lowest stair. The exercise is designed to wake up your glutes by flexing your hip joint. The step raises the foot off the ground, which encourages your hip flexion. As you bend and reach forward with your arms, you'll experience the glute lengthening. As you get to your end range of motion, which is the furthest point you can comfortably go, you'll naturally find yourself rocking back to the start position. You then go again. These movements are not to be held, like a stretch or a yoga pose. The idea is to gently move in and out of them, gradually increasing the range as you go.

1. Place one foot on a step and the other (the trailing foot) on the ground behind you, as in a stride.

2. Bend the knee of the front leg forward toward the toes. Avoid consciously controlling the movement of the knee, allow it to go where it comfortably wants to go, as you execute the movement. (Although the usual advice is to position the knee over the toe, Gary taught me that this actually limits our motion. Allowing it to follow the movements of the foot and hip is much more liberating for the body.)

3. As you bend the front knee, your hip will be drawn forward over the step toward the foot.

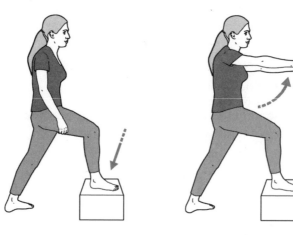

4. Gently reach out in front of you toward the horizon with your hands at hip height. As you move forward, the heel of the trailing foot will start to lift. This is perfectly normal.

5. As your hands reach forward at hip height, allow your upper body to follow as you attempt to reach as far as you comfortably can along this axis. (Your body should bend forward as a result of your hands reaching out.)

6. Our aim is to put most of our weight through the front foot on the step, with our hips sitting above the foot, and reaching forward with our arms, as in the picture.

7. As you become comfortable with this movement, and perhaps begin to find it easy, you can gradually lower your reach to knee height and out toward the horizon.

8. A long-term goal might be to safely place your fingertips on (or, ideally, beyond) the step. Do not hold these end positions but mindfully travel in and out of them back to upright.

9. Go as comfortably low as you feel is appropriate for you.

10. Repeat on the other leg.

For variation: Reach forward with only either the right or left hand to this position.

For progressions of this movement, please see the online videos at drchatterjee.com.

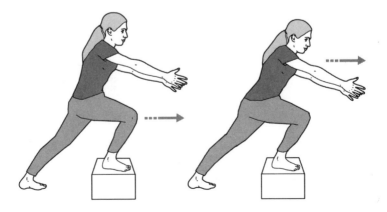

# MOVEMENT TWO: THE HIP ADDUCTION

This movement wakes the glute up in more than one way. It uses flexion, but it also uses the lateral motion of the hip. This is a whole body movement which targets the glutes and many other muscles which constitute the extensor chain.

1. Stand on a step.

2. Choose a leg to stand on.

3. While bending the knee of the standing leg, reach with the opposite foot behind and to the side, a bit like a curtsy, so that the toes of the reaching leg touch the floor.

4. Allow the weight-bearing knee to bend and to comfortably go where it wants. (Avoid consciously controlling the position of the knee.)

5. This begins to pull down the pelvis on the reaching-leg side and hike up the pelvis on the standing-leg side.

6. Raise the arm on the same side as your reaching leg and extend it toward the ceiling. When you reach high into your most comfortable end range, notice the stretch in that side of your abdomen.

7. You must maintain full weight bearing at all times on the standing leg. There is a temptation to put some weight on the reaching foot when it touches the floor. This should not happen—it should only tap the floor, not rest on it.

8. At your lowest comfortable point, bring yourself back up to standing and lower the opposite arm.

9. Allow both feet to rest on the step between repetitions of the same movement.

10. Change legs and repeat.

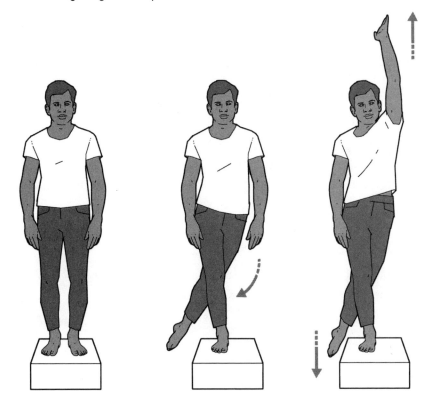

# MOVEMENT THREE: FOOT CLOCKS

Your glute movements are connected to the movement of your feet. Healthy foot motion naturally contributes to the glute lengthening in the correct way. This exercise will help make this happen. In addition you can start to identify "dark spaces" in your movement. These are the movements that your brain is not used to making. It's only by moving into these spaces that you can begin to reawaken pathways in your brain that have gone to sleep.

1. Start by standing with both feet together. Imagine yourself in the center of a large clock.

2. Relax the toes and choose a leg to stand on.

3. With the toes of the other leg, tap lightly at clock position 12 o'clock. Keep the tapping leg straight while allowing the standing leg to bend. The tapping leg should be stretched out as far as you can comfortably reach.

4. **After tapping, return to the start position.**

5. **Most of your weight should remain on the standing leg. This is the one that remains in the middle of the clock face.**

6. Allow the foot and knee of the standing leg to move freely as in the first two movements on the previous pages.

7. Begin a series of movements in which your reaching leg moves around the side of the clock that's the same side as your reaching leg (so, if standing on your right leg, follow the clock around from 12 counterclockwise to the left). Each time, ensure that the toes of the reaching leg only tap the floor lightly. The majority of your weight should remain on your standing leg.

8. Standing on your right leg aim to get as far around as 7 with the left leg (12, 11, 10, 9, 8, 7). Return to the start position before reaching to the next number on the clock face. Repeat this sequence between five and ten times.

9. Standing on your left leg aim to get as far around as 5 with the right leg (12, 1, 2, 3, 4, 5). Then go back to the start position. Repeat this sequence between five and ten times.

10. As the knee of your standing leg bends, and your other foot moves, your glutes will be encouraged to work.

11. Your focus is on the standing leg as the muscles react to the knee bending, the hip flexing and the foot flattening. The further you reach with your tapping leg, the more you will be activating your glutes.

12. Ensure that you work both legs.

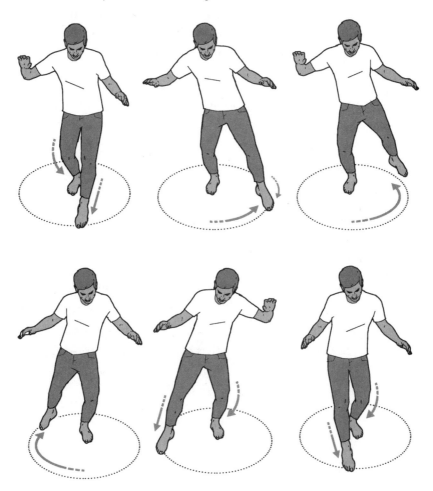

# MOVEMENT FOUR: 3D HIP EXTENSION

This movement puts all the joints in the body into a position that gives the glutes no option but to be fully activated. The front leg will experience the lengthening of its corresponding glute while the back leg will experience a full glute shortening. Working both sides means you'll be able to experience the full range of motion for both glutes.

1. Start by standing with your feet hip-width apart.

2. Place one foot forward at a comfortable distance. This distance will vary between individuals and you will need to do some experimentation. Start with a distance of 20 inches between the back foot big toe and the front foot one.

3. Relax the toes.

4. Bend the knee of your front foot while allowing the heel of the back foot to come up off the floor. You should keep the toes of the back foot on the ground.

5. Your weight should be mostly on the front foot. Try to let your pelvis move forward and come over your front foot.

6. Your torso should remain upright.

7. Try to think about your body moving forward and not down. This is not a gym-type lunge.

8. Keep the back knee straight and gently rotate it outward, without bending it, while keeping the back toes pointing straight forward.

9. The idea is to keep your head over your ribcage, your ribcage over your pelvis, and your pelvis over your front foot—so you're all nice and stacked. If you feel any pressure in your lower back it's likely you're not achieving this.

10. Raise both arms toward the ceiling.

11. Return to the starting position. Do this between five and ten times on each leg.

When you become comfortable with this movement, try one of the multiple progressions shown at drchatterjee.com.

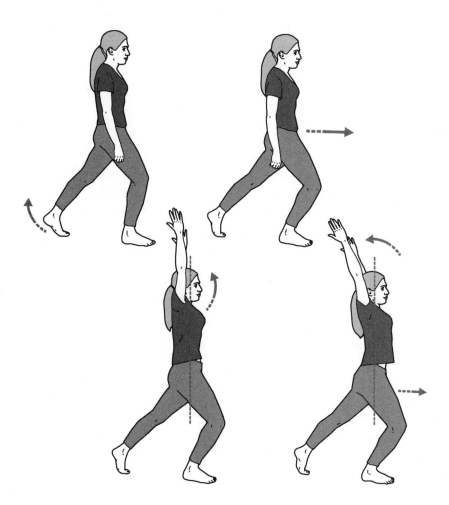

## TIPS TO WAKE UP YOUR GLUTES

My recommendation is that you do *at least* one of these four movements every single day. Once you know what you're doing, they don't take long. Any one of them can take under a minute. What's more, these are not gym-style exercises that will get you all sweaty. You don't need to change clothes, you don't need to schedule them in, they won't make you lose your breath. It's crucially important to keep reminding your body that it should be switching your glutes on and the best part is, it takes hardly any time or effort at all.

I do these exercises every single morning, while my coffee's brewing, in order to prepare my body for the day ahead. If you can fit in all four of them in a quick five-minute morning movement session, all of your subsequent movements throughout the day will be more efficient and more in harmony with the way your body is designed to move. Try to do the whole series at least four times per week.

Note: If you have any concerns whatsoever about performing any of the suggested movements in this pillar, you should consult a healthcare professional beforehand.

# SLEEP

We're in the middle of a sleep deprivation epidemic. We not only have far too many distractions in our daily lives but we also live in a "sleep is for wimps" culture that associates this natural and critical bodily function with laziness. Scientists from Oxford University claim we're getting between one and two hours less sleep per night than we did sixty years ago. In the context of an eight-hour sleep cycle, that's a hugely significant drop of up to 25 percent. Want to know how damaging this is? It's actually possible to put a number on at least one aspect of it. Sleep deprivation is thought to cost the British economy about £40 billion (about $55 billion) a year.

But this is a problem that goes far beyond financial cost. It's actively dangerous. Every time we drive when we're sleep deprived we're putting lives at risk. Recently I spent some time at a specialist center in Guildford, UK, to see this for myself. Using a simulator, the test subject drove the same route three times—first under normal conditions, then after drinking enough alcohol to remain just under the drink-and-drive cutoff, and finally when he had been restricted to having only three hours' sleep. When tired following his sleep restriction, he took up to four seconds to react to a hazard! This was a far worse result than when he'd had a drink. What I saw that day backs up a classic study from 1997 from the Queen Elizabeth Hospital in South Australia. The authors concluded that "relatively moderate levels of fatigue impair performance to an extent equivalent to or greater than is currently acceptable for alcohol intoxication." While this in itself is extremely worrying, what sleep researchers find particularly dangerous is that many sleep-deprived individuals don't even realize they're fatigued, and their performance impaired. Their perception is that they're doing very well.

But who isn't guilty of cutting corners on their sleep? I see it all the time with my patients and I've done it myself. When I'm feeling tired on the sofa in the evening, it's so tempting to keep watching television, or mindlessly surf the internet rather than making an active decision to fall asleep. You know the score . . . and so do I. But as I've immersed myself in sleep research over the past few years, I've changed the priority I give to sleep. It's no exaggeration to describe the results as life-changing. I feel happier, stronger and more alert, and my productivity has improved significantly.

The legendary sleep researcher Dr. Allan Rechtschaffen once wrote,

*"If sleep does not serve an absolutely vital function, then it is the biggest mistake the evolutionary process ever made."*

I love that quote because it really captures something not only about the vastness of sleep but also of its mystery. Scientists are still teasing out some highly significant aspects of exactly what happens when we sleep, and there's still much we don't know. All animals sleep, and the consequences of not doing so can be drastic. Rats deprived of their shut-eye die within a month. The longest any human has managed to stay awake is a mere eleven days. When seriously sleep deprived, people usually hallucinate and can even have fits. The fact that we spend a third of our entire lives asleep just hints at how critical it is for both our mental and physical well-being. Getting sufficient high-quality sleep is essential for the proper functioning of our minds and bodies. It's a core physiological process that many of us inadvertently regard as optional. Professor Matt Walker at the University of California, Berkeley, says, "There is no tissue within the body and no process within the brain that is not enhanced by sleep, or demonstrably impaired when you don't get enough."

# I

## SELF

# 1

## *Take Time to Sharpen the Saw*

If you were guaranteed that by using one hour a day in a particular way you would both enjoy and be more productive in the other twenty-three hours, would you do it? "Of course I would," you say.

But would you? You should, because it's literally true and can be proven by any individual willing to give it a fair trial.

The purpose and content of this one hour is to sharpen our three instruments—our body, our mind, and our spirit. It takes time and effort to sharpen them, but this time is negligible compared to the time (and nerves) saved.

Sometimes when we are terribly busy and under a lot of pressure, with many commitments and involvements, we become neglectful of the only instruments or tools we have to do our work. We think we haven't time to consider them. In a sense we are literally saying, "I am too busy sawing to take time to sharpen the saw."

I suggest three activities for this hour: one physical, one mental, one spiritual.

### *First, physical exercise.*

I won't take time to repeat all the obvious benefits of physical exercise but will only underscore the well-attested fact that a program of regular exercise increases one's efficiency in every facet of life, including the depth and restfulness of sleep. And the time taken can be minimal; just a few minutes of calisthenics and running in place in one's room or jogging around the yard or block is often sufficient. Exercising doesn't *take* time. It *saves* time. Still, few consistently do it.

### Second, planning.

Many of us feel that no matter how hard we apply ourselves or how we reorganize our time, we still have the feeling of being behind, of being pushed and pressured, of having more things to do than we can satisfactorily handle.

Sometimes the answer is found in working longer and harder, but often the real key is in working smarter.

To work smarter requires planning. Planning is creative thinking. It involves analyzing the needs of situations, setting goals or objectives, and determining a course of action in achieving them.

Such hard mental work takes a little time, but without it we become bogged down in detail and trivia, pushed here and there, responding only to the immediate pressures, to the demands and wants of others, to symptoms rather than to the causes of problems and the real needs of situations. Goethe put it this way: "Things which matter most must never be at the mercy of things which matter least." Careful planning helps us maintain a sense of perspective, of purpose, and of ordered priorities.

The more rushed we are, the more time we better spend planning our time and actions. Otherwise we become like the frantic driver who is too much in a hurry to go two miles out of his way to take the freeway and who then proceeds to burn himself up, rushing, then cussing every red light and every slowpoke on the old highway.

### Third, meditation, scripture study, and prayer.

Interwoven with planning is the effort to provide nourishment for the spirit, which we are all in constant need of as much as we need food for the body.

Prayerfully studying God's word in the scriptures and listening, through quiet meditation, to the still small voice within will result in a sense of eternal perspective, of divine need and purpose. It will also chasten, enlighten, and motivate, and is excellent preparation for secret prayer. Such prayer, offered from a sincere heart, is a perfect time for recommitment, for promising to obey the laws upon which the blessings requested are predicated. ". . . thy vows shall be offered up in righteousness on all days and at all times. . . ." (D&C 59:11.)

The great reformer Martin Luther understood this principle: "I've got so much to do today I'll need to spend another hour on my knees." To him prayer was not a mechanical duty but rather a source of power in releasing and multiplying his energies, by renewing an alliance with One who alone could make him equal to the day's tasks.

To use a physical analogy, such an alliance that is continually renewed in prayer is comparable to a farmer's using a powerful harvesting machine as contrasted to his neighbor's doing it all by hand because he couldn't "afford the time or money or bother" to rent one.

These three activities need not take more than one hour a day, but they will immeasurably influence the quality of the other twenty-three, for we are working upon the roots of both our problems and our successes. A sharp saw always cuts faster and better, and we must never be too busy to sharpen ours.

# 2

## *Be Strong in Hard Moments*

There are certain moments in every person's day that, if excellently used, will determine the direction and quality of all the other moments. These certain moments are few in number—sometimes very few. They are necessarily hard moments, testing moments.

Missionary work illustrates this well. There are generally three crucial moments in a missionary's day, and if he can be strong or true in these three hard moments, everything else tends to fall into place successfully.

These three moments are (1) getting up at 6:00 A.M.; (2) the initial moment of contacting; and (3) the moment when he gets an investigator to make a commitment.

1. The time of 6:00 A.M. in the schedule of missionary life symbolizes mastery over the flesh. Mind over mattress. If a missionary can overcome the pull of the flesh in the beginning moment of his day—often his hardest moment—he can overcome the lesser moments.

2. Initial contacting of new people takes initiative and courage. If the missionary will plunge into it at the appointed hour, refusing to shrink from it by doing easier things, he will develop power reserves to do many other hard things well.

3. Being strong, with love, in committing investigators to obey gospel laws, tests and nurtures both the emotional

and the spiritual roots of the missionary. Conducting safe but powerless philosophical gospel discussions takes little strength or courage.

Isn't it also true that if we, as parents or students, are courageous in just a few hard things each day, all else will fall into place? Sounds simple, I know, but I believe the answer is yes. The proof is in the doing, and this is not simple.

Certainly these things vary with each individual. Each must examine himself to find the few crucial daily moments that determine so much else.

Consider three things, three hard moments that are so basic and so determining for so many.

### First, getting up in the morning when we know we should.

Always being a few minutes behind in our work is a kind of emotional mortgage on the day. Tyrannized by the clock, we interpret almost every event selfishly. We fret and worry. We become overly impatient with weakness and mistakes, our own as well as those of others. Interruptions and inconveniences are resented. No time for kindness, for listening, for extra service. The spirit of rushing and hurrying destroys a good family spirit.

The consequences of a few minutes more sleep are often so exhausting!

### Second, making reconciliation to the Lord's will.

To reconcile means to bring together, to unite, to bring back into harmony and friendship. If we are not careful to daily drink of the "living waters," we can easily and slowly become strangers to the Lord and his ways and to our own divine identity and purpose. We learn his ways from prayerfully searching the scriptures. Listening then to the still small voice of conscience and then committing in secret prayer to obey its promptings that day complete this reconciliation.

### Third, to control our tongue.

To not say the unkind or critical thing, particularly when provoked and/or fatigued, is a supreme kind of self-mastery.

President McKay taught, "Never must there be expressed in a Latter-day Saint home an oath, a condemnatory term, an expression of anger or jealousy or hatred. Control it! Do not express it! You do what you can to produce peace and harmony no matter what you may suffer."

As in all things, the Savior is again the perfect model of this principle. Everything culminated in his supreme tests at Gethsemane and Calvary. We are all beneficiaries of his being strong and true in that transcendent moment of eternity.

To simply understand the pervasive power of a few moments in a day is highly motivating in itself, in marshaling and unifying our will, our nerve, and our energy.

Someone rightly defined courage as the quality of every quality at its highest testing point.

# 3

*Work on the Roots*

What would you think if a person were to construct a dam, for aesthetic reasons, on a mountain top instead of the base of a canyon?

Or what would you think if one were to attempt to build an internal combustion engine on the principle that gases contract when heated?

In either case you would answer that the individuals were ignoring basic natural laws: gravity and expansion of gas when heated. Neither the dam nor the engine would work, regardless of how beautifully located or well constructed.

These two farfetched examples illustrate a simple point: to make things work we must understand and work with, not against, the nature of things.

Actually, these examples are not so farfetched after all. The history of every field of science gives abundant evidence of how new scientific discoveries upturn and make obsolete many well-established theories and practices. Many of the great scientific breakthroughs have been breakwiths.

Take the applied science of medicine as another example. In tribal days witch doctoring was the accepted thing. The natives thought they understood the nature of things —that the evil spirits caused disease and that the witch doctor possessed magical powers. To them, these ideas or assumptions were facts. To us today these assumptions are superstitions, born of ignorance and fear. Pure research into the nature of things has enabled applied medical science to work seeming miracles, extending our life-span twice that of our forebears several generations ago.

This thinking has direct application to the fields of human behavior, such as family relations, communications, and leadership, for, as with the physical and medical science analogies, if our theories of reality (and we are all acting on them) aren't accurate, we're in trouble.

The vital question, therefore, is: What is the nature of things regarding man and his relationships?

Our answers come from basically two sources: man's discoveries and God's revelations. If these two ever seem to conflict, revelations must take precedence, for the tools of science are finite and cannot refute or explain the infinite.

To deny or to ignore what has been revealed about man doesn't change the nature of things one bit! It simply becomes another case of witch doctoring.

The following basic realities about man have been revealed and have profound, far-reaching consequences in our discussions of human relations.

1. Man is an immortal spirit, clothed in a physical body.

2. His growth and development are governed by spiritual and moral laws.

3. Through disobedience to those laws, man becomes insecure and alienated from himself, from his Creator, and from his fellowmen.

4. By obedience to the laws and ordinances of the gospel, through the atonement of Christ, man becomes secure and unified within himself, with his Creator, and with his fellowmen.

Based on the above analysis, I offer two personal convictions.

First, the real nature of our problems is spiritual.

That is, the roots of our problems lie in our disobeying natural laws—knowingly or unknowingly.

Examine any problems you face from that standpoint, whether family finances, relationship breakdowns between husband and wife or parent and child, fear of failure, obesity, confusion in making decisions, despair over world conditions, or whatever.

Start with the surface complaint and ask what caused it. Then ask what caused that and what caused that and so on. Such causal-chain thinking will eventually lead back to show either a lack of understanding of reality (life's purpose, man's nature, the governing laws) or a lack of commitment and self-discipline to live accordingly —thus procrastination, impatience, overeating, selfishness, etc.

Notice how most of these discussions eventually return to the fundamental principles of understanding or commitment or discipline, expressed in various ways.

Second, the basic solution to our problems also lies within ourselves. We can't escape the nature of things. Like it or not, realize it or not, God's authority is in us. That is, his nature, his laws, and our conscience.

It's futile to fight our battles on the wrong battlefields. We must work on causes, not symptoms. Taking aspirin for a headache won't eliminate future headaches.

The spiritual resources available to us are fathomless and possess infinite wisdom and power. But the initiative, the first step, lies with us.

"For every thousand hacking at the leaves of evil, there is one striking at the root." (Thoreau.)

# 4

## *The Power of Self-Understanding*

One of the principal reasons we have a hard time understanding others is because we lack understanding of ourselves.

A little thinking will reveal why this is so. The very tool we use to understand another is within us, and if we are confused about ourselves—the lens we look through—obviously, inevitably, we will also be cloudy about others.

In light of this idea, study the following story of a woman who came to better understand her family problems and who changed her life through gaining precious insights about herself and acting on them.

"For years and years I fought with my children and they fought with each other. I was constantly judging and criticizing and scolding.

"I knew something had to be done. But I didn't know what. I did know my incessant critical nagging was hurting their self-esteem and the whole spirit of our home, causing much of the contention.

"Again and again I would resolve and try to change. And just as often I would fall back. Then I'd feel awful—guilty—angry with myself. I hated myself, and as I saw my own weaknesses in my children's behavior, I took out my self-anger on them. Then I'd feel more guilty, and the more guilt I felt the more anger I expressed.

"Eventually I decided to make my problems a matter of sustained and specific and earnest prayer. Gradually I came to two insights about my real motives and reasons for my negative critical behavior.

"First, I came to see more clearly the impact of my own childhood home experiences. Our home was broken in almost every way and eventually ended in divorce. I can't ever remember seeing my parents talk through their problems and differences. They would either argue and fight or they'd angrily separate. The silent treatment —sometimes for days.

"So when I had to deal with the same issues and problems with my own family, I had no model or example to follow. I really didn't know what to do. Instead of finding a model or fighting it through within myself, I'd take out my confusion and frustration on the kids. And yet, as much as I didn't like it, I found myself dealing with my children just as my parents did with us.

"One more immensely helpful self-insight came to me. I was trying to win, to wrest social approval out of my own children's behavior. Because I was constantly fearful of being embarrassed, I constantly instructed and threatened and bribed and manipulated to get my kids to be-have—all so others would think well of me.

"I could then see, in my own hunger for approval, that I was shielding my own children from growth and responsibility. I was helping cause the very thing I feared the most—irresponsible behavior."

I asked this woman how these two self-insights helped her.

She answered, "They've made all the difference in the world. I now realize I have to conquer my own problems within myself instead of taking them out on others.

"My unhappy, confused childhood inclined me to be negative but it didn't force me. I still had my agency. I could choose to respond differently. It was futile to blame my parents or my circumstances.

"Oh, it was hard to admit this to myself—very hard!

I struggled with years of accumulated pride. But once I swallowed the bitter pill, I had a marvelously free feeling. I was in control. I could choose a better way. I was responsible for myself.

"I've now learned to retire frequently to myself and win my own battles privately, to get my motives straight. And now when I get into a frustrating situation I stop. I pause. I back away from impulsively speaking or striking out. I try for perspective and control. Sometimes I simply go alone and struggle the thing through on my own. I find new models, new examples to follow, the perfect one being the Savior. The scriptures and prayer have helped greatly."

Look at the miracles these two self-insights produced! This woman's new understanding of herself taught her how to use it to control herself. It also inspired her to take responsibility for her own behavior and attitudes, for both her actions and her reactions.

We simply do not win our own battles on someone else's battlefield.

"The greatest battles of life are fought out daily in the silent chambers of the soul." (David O. McKay.)

Private victories precede public victories.

# 5

## *Patience: Its Nature and Its Growth*

Many admit to being impatient. "I have some virtues but patience isn't one of them. I wish I could develop more patience," we say.

Not knowing exactly how to develop patience, we generally forget about it and go about our lives in the spirit of rush and hurry, critical of the slowness and weaknesses of others. Then, in times of stress, particularly around loved ones, our impatient mood surfaces and our temper flashes. We may say something we don't really mean or intend to say—all out of proportion to reality.

Or we may become sullen, slowly burning inside and communicating through emotion and attitude, rather than words, eloquent messages of criticalness, judgment, and rejection. Our harvest is bitter: hurt feelings, strained relationships, little growth. Again seeing the fruits of our impatience, we repeat, "I wish I were more patient," almost as if this were a quirk of our nature we could do nothing about.

Let's examine two questions: What is patience? and How can we develop it?

1. Notice how literally patience is the practical expression of faith, hope, wisdom, and love. First, patience is not a passive virtue as some think. Patience is extremely active emotionally.

For instance, what kind of father would slap or criticize or otherwise punish his infant son when he totters and falls while learning to walk? Why is this extreme foolishness so self-evident to us? Because we all know that falling is part of learning to walk. We know if we punish falling, the boy will stop trying. Unless he tries he'll never learn to walk. He'll just crawl.

This simple analogy can be extended to include all learning and development. Patience accepts the reality of life that in all things there is a process, a step one, step two, step three process that cannot be ignored or bypassed.

Faith embodies patience. It is a contradiction for someone to think or feel he has faith but lacks patience. Faith deals with the unseen. The father helps and encourages his tottering son to walk. Why? Because of what he sees? No, for he sees only falling. He does it because of what he does not see, because of what he believes. He believes in his son's potential to walk and he acts accordingly. That's faith. It's also hope. That's why he patiently encourages and waits.

Patience obviously, therefore, is not indifference, is not sullen endurance, is not a matter of doing nothing. Patience is faith in action. Patience is emotional diligence.

Consider the scriptural definition of patience: long-suffering. We suffer inside when we want something now and can't have it. We suffer inside when we have to wait for someone to bungle through the learning process to do their job. "It's easier to do it myself," we reason. We suffer inside when the results we want, and are judged by, require the willing cooperation of those who either don't know how or don't care.

The willingness to suffer inside so others can grow takes love. As we become aware of our suffering, we learn about ourselves and our own motives and weaknesses. Knowledge of ourselves and life's processes, combined with self-restraint, produces the sense and ability to know when to do what. This is wisdom.

What a small price such long-suffering is for such

huge gains! "Patience is bitter but its fruit is sweet." (Rousseau.)

2. The development of patience is akin to the development of one's body or muscles through resistance exercises. In exercising, a point is reached when the strain on the muscle causes its fiber to rupture. Then when nature repairs the broken fiber, she overcompensates and the muscle grows in strength, elasticity, and power.

Similarly, there are three aspects in the development of patience fiber.

First, purpose and a commitment to it. Those who would like more patience but lack a strong desire and sense of purpose (the *way* of it) will be easily uprooted under the first strain.

Second, resistance. Patience is not developed as knowledge is acquired from books, but only under testing and strain. Life provides abundant opportunities to practice patience—to stretch the emotional fiber—from waiting for a late person or plane to listening quietly to your child's feelings and experiences when other things are pressing. Cheerfully bearing the little annoyances and trials of every day builds and strengthens the emotional fiber for times of real stress and calamity.

Third, be patient with the development of patience itself. Otherwise, you'll give up on both the effort and yourself. The roots of impatience lie in other weaknesses and habits and are not pulled up without some pain and consistent effort through time. Have faith in your own unseen potential.

# 6

## *Three Processes:*
## *Knowing, Choosing, Doing*

The most spectacular and celebrated—and certainly the most involving—technical achievement of all time was the Apollo 11 moon trip. How ironic to witness such herculean feats while fighting hot and cold wars all around this globe. As one observer put it, "We are technical giants and moral pigmies."

Why? Why such a massive gap between our technical and our human relationship achievements? Many think it is because the physical sciences have outstripped the social sciences and therefore we need to pour more of our energies and resources into the study of how to improve human relationships. I believe this idea is not only false but highly misleading.

If we include the teachings of the Lord, the social or human behavior sciences are far ahead of the physical sciences. The basic principles and laws given have never been improved upon or changed since Adam, the first man. Founded on the Ten Commandments, they move to the Golden Rule and the laws of love, repentance, and forgiveness.

This is not so with the physical sciences. Much that was taught as scientific fact in school years ago is discarded today. Many of the great "breakthroughs" were "break-withs."

Where, then, is the lag? In doing. In applying. The applied social sciences lag far behind the applied physical sciences.

Each of us can look about our own lives to see the evidence and the origin of this gap between knowing and doing. Few of us "do" as well as we "know." Why is this so? I suggest the answer lies in our skipping or neglecting a fundamental connecting step or link between what we know and what we do. This is the step or process of choosing.

Choosing means to pause and stand back for perspective, to think deeply, and then to decide our own actions and reactions. Choosing means to accept responsibility for ourselves and our attitudes, to refuse to blame others or circumstances.

Choosing, then, means to commit ourselves strongly to that which we decide to do. This committing process often involves a real internal struggle, ultimately between competing motives or between conflicting concepts of ourselves.

This choosing (deciding and committing) step can break the binding power of habits if enough effort goes into it. This is more than strong resolution or sheer willpower. Many exert great willpower to overcome a fault or habit or to accomplish an important project, but they don't inwardly believe they will really succeed. They see themselves, perhaps unconsciously, as incapable or unworthy of success. They've failed before—they'll fail again. So before the doing process begins, they are already defeated. Private defeats precede public defeats.

This choosing process, therefore, also involves "belief power" (meaning great mental exertion)—seeing and imagining and feeling ourselves successfully doing what we desire to. Such a believing process welds the conscious and the unconscious forces together.

We have all experienced something powerful "connect" within ourselves once we made our mind up on a matter. We simply knew we could and would do it. And we did it. The private victory preceded the public victory.

In this choosing opportunity rests man's free agency—his supreme unique gift—and his accountability. Through it, man alone can use and build on the accumulated knowledge of the ages. No animal can do this. Through it, man alone can break with the past, even deeply imbedded habits, and determine his own future. No animal can do this. Deterministic philosophy—the idea that biological heritage and/or social environment sets or determines man's character and conduct—is animal psychology.

But unless we realize both our free agency and our power to choose and then use them wisely, our actions will be determined by the conditions, within and without, of our lives.

Look at it this way. Unless the choosing gear connects knowing to doing, we will still be connected to old habit gears and/or to the gears of others and of circumstances.

This choosing process takes time and great mental and spiritual exertion. Prayer and ordinance work can serve this purpose magnificently and release great powers, within and without. We'll do what we know we should if we regularly covenant deep enough to do so.

# 7

## *Distinguish Between Person and Performance*

Parents, teachers, and leaders frequently bemoan the power that acceptance and popularity by the peer group have over their youth. "What can we do to decrease its influence and increase our own?" they plead.

There is, I believe, a common denominator behind much of the behavior of youth, an understanding of which is immensely helpful in dealing with them. It has to do with what is the primary source of their security or sense of worth.

Consider two terms—intrinsic and extrinsic—and the subsequent reasons. *First, intrinsic.* This means that one's primary source of security or sense of worth lies within. One has worth apart from his performance and apart from others' opinions of him. He feels deep inside, without having to think about it, "I'm good. I'm of worth, in and of myself."

Such a person possesses the inner strength and courage to act on what he knows is right regardless of popularity. In his own eyes he is somebody and stands for something, so social pressure, even rejection, doesn't control him or "wipe him out."

*Second, extrinsic.* This means that one's primary sense of worth and value lies outside himself, particularly in the opinion of other people.

Again, it isn't so much an intellectual matter as it is emotional. This person may think "I am a child of God" but not feel it. His sense of goodness lies almost entirely in the good he does, not in the good he is.

Consequently, lacking security within, he seeks it without—sometimes almost desperately in trying to be all things to all people.

Policed by the reactions of others, he's torn inside as he finds everyone expects different things: "My parents expect this, the Church that, and my friends that." Confused and lonely, he often withdraws into a "safe" world of his own making.

Perhaps a more typical reaction pattern with many youth is to conform to the values and expectations of the group from which they seek acceptance and approval, and to rebel, to greater or lesser degrees, against their parents and their parents' values. The first outward manifestations of this rebellion to conformity may be dress and hair styles, language used, and defensive attitudes. It will often lead to other compromises—vulgarity, lying, cheating, stealing, and eventually smoking, drinking, drugs, unchastity. Then, of course, these perversions of life horribly compound and complicate both the root problems and the way back.

Our efforts to reach them, to reclaim them, are sometimes done in the very way (judging, moralizing) they interpret as rejection of them as persons, exalting again only the good they should do. This solidifies both their rebellious patterns and their present loyalties as the only source of their identity or sense of being a person, an individual.

In some way we need to communicate an understanding and acceptance of them as persons without approving or condoning their behavior. Although difficult to do, it can be done. Our youth want it more than they would dare tell us.

One of the basic early causes of extrinsic sense of worth is the widespread tendency at home and school and in society to compare one person with another and, most importantly, to emotionally reward (praise, warmth, love) and punish (impatience, displeasure, judgment, rejection) on the basis of that comparison.

Think this through carefully: when comparisons are habitual, when a person's worth and his performance are one and the same thing, gradually the source of worth moves out of him (intrinsic) and into someone else's opinion (extrinsic) of his performance. "She's our bright one." "He's the slow one." "He's smart but he just won't apply himself like his brother." "I just can't understand it at all—you should have done better than Susan." "Your grades are getting embarrassing to us, honey."

Such labels or definitions habitually given are soon believed and lived up to and emotionally accepted as part of a person's concept of self. "Of course I failed—'cause I'm a failure. Just ask anybody."

It is vital to distinguish between a person and his behavior or performance. While we need to disapprove of bad behavior and reward superior performance, we first need to communicate and help build in our young people a sense of intrinsic worth and goodness and esteem totally apart from these comparisons and judgments. Ironically, success in doing this will powerfully serve to inspire superior effort. It is a self-fulfilling prophecy.

The very power to understand the crucial distinction between person and performance and to communicate intrinsic worth to others flows naturally out of our own sense of intrinsic worth and value. Otherwise we will find ourselves wresting our own personal security from the performance of our youth and will therefore be unable to communicate intrinsic worth to them.

# 8

## *Eight Sources of Inner Security*

When a person has a deep inner sense of personal worth, he is more effective in all phases of his life. He is also genuinely happy for the successes of others, feeling that nothing is being taken from him.

Consider eight different, although interrelated, sources of a deep sense of intrinsic worth and inner personal security. Carefully notice how the items emphasized, under each of the eight sources, deal with developing a sense of worth within each individual, rather than without, from opinions or comparisons.

### *First, the family.*

One's emotional roots lie primarily in the unconditional love and regard that parents have for their children and for each other. Frequently, time is taken for each one for private visits and understanding. When one parent shows kindness, respect, and courtesy to the other parent, the children feel value is also given to them—intrinsic value.

Family councils are held. Each opinion is listened to, respected, and considered. There's an absence of comparing one against another, of arbitrary rule making, of inconsistent mood-of-the-moment disciplining. There's the presence of family prayer, family traditions, family goals, schedules, duties, limits, rules, rights, privileges, consistently firm and fair discipline, honoring of promises.

"There is beauty all around when there's love at home."

### Second, church activity and service.

Condemning the sin, yet valuing the sinner, the Church places supreme value on the intrinsic worth of each individual. Whenever we reach outside ourselves in the Lord's pattern to serve another, we communicate value to him and receive value in return. Genuine involvement ("with real intent") in teaching, leading, ordinance work for the living or the dead, or merely attending and participating in the church climate yields a sense of individual worth and personal security.

### Third, nature.

Nature is very life-affirming and bequeaths its silent strength to one who takes time to feel and to appreciate. To absorb ourself in the magnificent beauty of the mountains, to spend time at the beach or in any lovely natural setting, including our own backyard, brings an intrinsic sense of worth, if we take the time to be still and to meditate, to drink it all in.

### Fourth, continuing education.

Education's main value does not lie in getting knowledge, much of which will be obsolete sooner or later. It certainly doesn't lie in credits earned or degrees conferred. These may open doors of opportunity, but only real competence will keep them open. In fact, in our rapidly changing world there is no "future," no economic security in any job or situation. The only real economic security lies within the person, in his competence and power to produce.

Education's main value lies in learning how to continually learn, how to think and to communicate, how to appreciate and to produce, how to adapt to changing realities without sacrificing changeless values. Result? An inner confidence in the basic ability to cope successfully with whatever life brings.

To keep informed and alive, adults need some kind of system that contains balance and substance and requires mental concentration and discipline—a reading program, discussion groups, a correspondence course, an education week, or whatever.

Children need to be encouraged to be conscientious on a daily basis in their school and homework. Value should be placed on their disciplined efforts and love of learning and creativity as well as on grades and other academic achievements. Youth really know inside how they're doing in school, in several important ways, far more than their teachers or parents do, and their own honest self-evaluations should be discussed and respected.

### Fifth, anonymous service.

Whenever we do good for others when no one knows save God and us alone, our intrinsic sense of worth and respect increases. ". . . thy Father which seeth in secret himself shall reward thee openly." (Matt. 6:4.)

### Sixth, daily work.

Doing ordinary everyday work well brings its own rewards to each person. But doing it excellently, going the second mile, doing something creative and unique multiplies those intrinsic rewards. Two activities in work will influence results the most: planning and honest two-way communication with key people. A personal sense of self-mastery is internally more rewarding than any form of economic or social reward.

### Seventh, a spiritually rich private life.

Daily and weekly immersion in gospel teachings, in the scriptures, in private worship, in meditation and prayer releases enormous resources within us of peace and serenity, understanding and courage. The scriptures teach that we will abide in the Lord's love—the perfect source of divine definition of self—if we abide in his word.

### Eighth, integrity.

When we live true to the light and truth we have re-

ceived, we will receive more light and truth. If we are un-
true to that light (our conscience), we experience disunity
and insecurity within. Then, unless we repent, this internal
warring will breed guilt, anger, and defensiveness, and will
undermine both our resolve and our capacity to tap the
other seven sources of personal security.

The key is to be a doer, not just a hearer; to be a
light, not a judge of the darkness.

# 9

## *True Freedom Lies Within*

The ultimate, perhaps the last, freedom is the right and power to decide within how anybody or anything outside ourself will affect us. Many people are simply unaware they have this capacity, this freedom.

During a speech on this subject once a woman in the audience literally lit up. She seemed so ecstatic and radiant she could hardly contain herself. At the conclusion of the talk I went to her and asked what had happened. She answered, "You have no idea what the point on attitude control means to me. You see, I have been a full-time nurse for over three years to the most miserable, ungrateful, crotchety old man you can imagine. But up until tonight I have been feeling how miserable he has made my life. Tonight I have come to realize that I have chosen to be miserable. He hasn't made me miserable. I have chosen to respond to his behavior in that way. This is a bitter pill to swallow. But the thing that really hit home to me was the thought that since I had freely chosen the negative response to a negative situation, I have the freedom to choose otherwise. No longer will he control my disposition. I will control it."

Dr. Viktor E. Frankl, a Jewish Austrian psychotherapist, was imprisoned in various concentration camps in Germany during the second world war. His parents, his brother, and his wife died in the camps or were sent to the gas ovens. Except for his sister, his entire family perished in these camps. He was stripped of all his possessions. He suffered torture and innumerable indignities. He never knew from one moment to the next if his path would lead to the gas chambers or the ovens, or if he would be among the "saved" who would remove the bodies or shovel out the ashes of those so fated.

One day, alone in a small room, stripped naked, he began to become aware of the last freedom. It was the only freedom, he said, they could not take from him: he could decide within himself how all of this was going to affect him. He proceeded to act upon this awareness. It grew and grew through mental concentration and self-discipline until he acquired unusual controls within himself. He became an inspiration to those around him, even to the guards. He helped others find meaning in their suffering and dignity in their prison existence.

The essence of the Savior's life and teachings deals with internal freedom or control: turn the other cheek, go the second mile, "pray for those who curse you," "love your enemies," etc. The Lord told the Prophet Joseph Smith that his suffering "shall give thee experience, and shall be for thy good." This very kind of internal attitude control, this freedom, provides the most powerful evidence of overcoming the world and of one's true discipleship to the Son of God.

The world's doctrine of determinism links stimulus and response together as inseparable. However, once we are aware that we can decide within ourself what our response will be to a given stimulus (environment or person), they become separated. This very awareness becomes the embryo of our freedom. If we then continue to act on that awareness by overcoming evil with good, by returning cheerfulness in the face of gloom and pessimism, patience toward the impatient, kindness to the unkind, our internal freedom will continue to grow and grow. It is exactly because we have this freedom that we are responsible and will be held responsible by its author, our Creator.

For our purpose here, let us define liberty as the opportunity in life to choose between alternatives and freedom as the internal power or capacity to choose between alternatives. In this sense Dr. Frankl had freedom but not liberty. Similarly we may have liberty (opportunity) but not freedom (power), perhaps because of our addiction to the habit of gratifying an appetite or passion.

For instance, in sports, a golfer studies each situation and uses the appropriate club. He has freedom (developed power). But if he only knows how to use one club, although he could choose others, he has no power (freedom).

So in our relations with others. If we are addicted to interpret every situation in terms of our own convenience or pleasure or ego and then become upset or angry when things don't go our way, we truly are slaves, even as we proclaim our freedom to do our "own thing."

Therefore, freedom is responsible self-discipline, the opposite of license. We act from divine principles and conscience within rather than react to changing and fickle values and realities without.

# 10

## *Step-by-Step Victory Over Self*

Most relationship problems stem from personal problems, in at least two distinct ways.

First is the way we take out our guilt on others. When we are not true to our conscience, we are at war with ourselves. Rather than repenting, the natural tendency is to take that war out on others. We do it when we find their weakness, the mote in their eye, and thus can momentarily forget the beam in our own—mote-beam sickness.

Much of the arguing, contending, and criticizing in family circles follows a combination of low achievement and high fatigue. As one put it, "When I don't feel good about myself, you better watch out!"

The second kind of personal problem is interwoven with the first and perhaps is its prime cause—a lack of self-discipline. When we are controlled by our appetites and passions, we inevitably have relationship problems. All it takes is a time of stress and/or fatigue to uproot our best intentions.

The following true story is one clear illustration of how relationships inevitably deteriorate through a lack of self-discipline and how they can be made beautiful by growth in self-discipline, which I'm defining here as the ability to make and keep promises.

It involves an undisciplined missionary who pleaded with his mission president for a transfer from his companion, claiming, "We just can't get along." The president counseled him that he could learn to get along if he would only hold his tongue, serve his companion, and obey true principles of self-control, of love and service. The missionary resolved to do so but his hair-trigger temper gripped him more than his resolve. As with many, he had the habit of making and breaking resolutions.

Again and again he requested a transfer, once saying, "I'm afraid of what I might do if I really lost my temper." And again and again his president would commit him to principles of self-control, of love and service. Nothing seemed to take until one day the leader realized that, in a sense, he was teaching him to run before he could walk, for his reactions and emotions were controlled far more by the habits and appetites of his flesh and the temper of his spleen than by the momentary sincerity of his resolves.

If hungry, he'd eat, and eat, and eat. If sleepy, he'd sleep—even in meetings. If upset, he'd show it. If angry, he'd express it. Yet, when he felt fine, he was ever so sweet and pleasant and ever so repentant and resolved. He merely took the course of least resistance in each situation.

So, one day, after weeks of counseling, the leader asked the missionary to promise to get up at 5:55 A.M. for one month.

"I can't understand it," he retorted. "I asked you to help me with my relationship problem and you ask me to get up at 5:55."

"Elder, how can you possibly control and direct your emotions until you have more control of the very instrument through which you express your emotions—your body? Let's begin at the first step and take one at a time. Will you get up at 5:55 for one full month?"

"I'm not sure I can."

"Then don't promise to. Will you for a week?"

"I will," he answered.

A week later: "Did you keep your promise?"

"I did."

"Congratulations! Now let's take step two. Will you study alone and with your companion for two and one half hours every morning for a week?"

"I can't. My mind jumps all around the place."

"Will you just sit there for two and a half hours and try?"

"I will."

He did it. Week by week, month by month, he made and kept promises. Little by little, line upon line, he grew in self-mastery, in integrity, in spirituality. His relationships with others, even with difficult persons, were magnificent, and he became one of the most powerful and effective and respected missionary leaders in the field. Through making and keeping small resolves, small promises, he had won a victory over himself. He learned the hard way that "the body is a good servant but a bad master."

There are several principles of personal growth and human relations here. Consider five, which build on each other.

1.  We must never make a promise we will not keep.

2.  To grow we must make promises (resolutions, commitments, oaths, covenants) to do better, to be better.

3.  We must use self-knowledge and be very careful and selective about the promises we make, for all things must be done in order (in the right sequence).

4.  Our ability to make and keep promises is the measure of our faith in ourselves and of our integrity.

5.  This integrity, or self-mastery, is also basic to our faith in God, for his promises to us are conditioned on our keeping our promises to him.

Therefore, in one sense, the whole system of relationships—human and divine—is based on a step-by-step victory over self.

"A 1,000-mile journey begins with a single step."

# II

# RELATIONSHIPS

# 11

# *How to Influence Others*

The accompanying diagram shows how one can effectively influence others. It will help to refer to it as you consider the subsequent reasoning together with the real human influence problems and challenges you face.

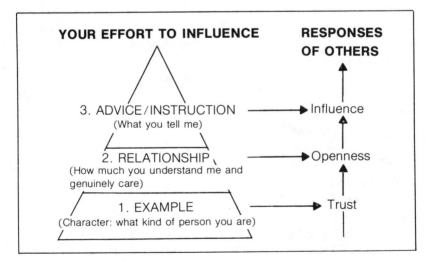

First, note the three basic interrelated phases or levels: (1) example, (2) relationship, and (3) advice/instruction. To illustrate how each phase necessarily builds on the other, assume for a moment I am the person—your spouse or child or worker or boss or neighbor or whoever—you are attempting to influence, perhaps after some past failure to do so.

1. *"The key and foundation to your influence with me is your example, your actual conduct,"* I begin. *"Your example flows naturally out of your character or the kind of a person you truly are, not what others say you are or what you may want me to think you are; it is evidenced in how I actually experience you.*

*"Your essential character is constantly radiating, communicating. From it in the long run, I come to instinctively trust or distrust you and your efforts with me. It is a matter of degree, of course.*

*"If your life runs hot and cold, if you're both caustic and kind and, above all, if your private performance doesn't square with your public performance, it's very hard for me to open up with you. Then as much as I may want and even need to receive your love and influence, I don't feel safe enough to expose my opinions and experiences and my tender feelings. Who knows what will happen? I've been hurt before and I'm not going to chance it again."*

2. *"But unless I open up with you, unless you understand me and my unique situation and feelings, you won't know how to advise or counsel me. What you say is all good and fine, but you see, it doesn't quite pertain to me.*

*"You say you care about and appreciate me. (Oh, how I wish I could believe that!) But how could you appreciate when you don't even understand? Just words. I can't trust words. If you would just try to understand . . ."*

3. *"Unless you're influenced by my uniqueness, I'm not going to be influenced by your advice. I'm too angry and defensive—perhaps I'm too guilty and afraid—to be influenced, even though inside I know I need what you have to tell me. Besides, you don't even practice what you preach."*

In our attempts to influence others, we commonly make three kinds of mistakes, all related to either ignoring or shortcutting these same three intertwined phases of influence.

First, we try to tell or advise others before we have established any understanding relationship, any real communication. Our advice, however sound, will generally not be received until the feeling is good. I suggest the supreme skill needed here is empathy.

Second, we try to build or rebuild a relationship without making any fundamental change in our conduct or attitude. If our example is pockmarked with inconsistency and insincerity, no amount of win-friends-influence-people technique will work. As Emerson so aptly put it, "What you are shouts so loudly in my ears I can't hear what you say."

Third, we assume that a good example and a good relationship are sufficient, that we don't need to explicitly teach the "shoulds" of life. If this were true, we would need neither weekday school nor Sunday School.

We need to teach the words of life and of eternal life by both example and precept. We need to give the vision and to testify of it. Just as vision without love contains no motivation, so also love without vision contains no goals, no guidelines, no standards, no lifting power.

And realistically we need to focus others' attention on our Lord and Savior, the perfect exemplar, so as to gradually lessen their dependency on our imperfect examples (as was evidenced in the above monologue). As "the Way, the Life, and the Truth," he simultaneously embodies and integrates all three levels and is the perfect source and model of influence.

# 12

## *Give Positive Experiences*

One of the main reasons behind communication break-downs is because the people involved interpret the same event differently. Their different natures and different background experiences condition them to do so. If they then interact without taking into account why they see things differently, they begin to judge each other.

This judging tears at the relationship, compounding the communication breakdown and spawning longer-term personality conflicts.

For instance, take as small a thing as a difference in room temperature. The thermostat on the wall clearly registers 75 degrees. One complains "It's too hot," and opens the windows; the other complains "It's too cold," and closes them.

Who is right? Is it too hot or too cold? The fact is they are both right.

Can two people disagree and both be right? Obviously yes. Each is right from his own point of view. And probably each will respect this fact and either stop complaining or make a compromise satisfactory to both.

But what if they tried to prove each other wrong, saying such things as, "Too hot? Are you crazy? I'm freezing!"

Judging another's sanity or sincerity is a personal

attack and creates new and different relationship problems that are far more difficult to solve.

When we apply this same reasoning to the sense of seeing or to the sense of hearing, we open up a fruitful understanding of human problems.

We do this in the classroom with some simple pictures. First, we briefly show a picture of a young girl to one group and a picture of an old lady to another group. This first experience conditions how they will see and interpret the next experience. We then show both groups a composite picture, containing the outlines of both the young girl and the old woman. Finally, we ask them what they see and watch them interact with each other.

Several things inevitably happen. First, with few exceptions, they see as they were conditioned to—one group asserting "She's a young woman," and the other group answering "No, she's an old woman." Second, they begin to argue and frequently end in personally attacking either the judgment or the sincerity of the other. One says, "Don't put me on. You can see that wrinkled face and haggard old look just as well as I can!" The other answers, "Wrinkled face! What's wrong with you? She's lovely, young, and petite!" As each grows defensive he becomes even more convinced that "I'm right and you're wrong."

One person will eventually come to see another's point of view by first assuming that the other is sincere and then seeking to understand through asking and listening rather than telling and judging. Gradually, through respectful communication, almost everyone comes to see both points of view, usually with an "Oh! I see it!" Yet, I have students to this day who cannot. They invested so much ego in their defense as to freeze their initial perception or point of view.

The accompanying diagram attempts to summarize this most useful learning, which is applicable to every area of life, particularly the family.

While referring to the diagram, consider three implications:

1. Center blocks: Experiences tend to condition how

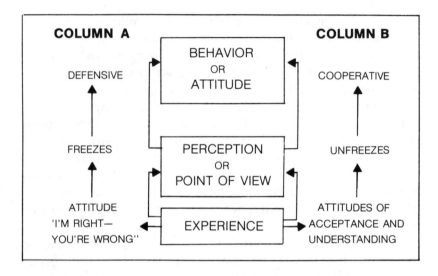

we perceive, and we behave accordingly—like looking at life through a very private lens or filter.

2. Column A: When we try to change another's behavior or attitude by telling and by judging ("I'm right—you're wrong"), we ignore implication No. 1 and thus give an experience that tends to freeze or reinforce his intial perception and also to increase his defensiveness.

3. Column B: When we assume the other is right from his point of view (for he is!) and then try to understand his point of view by asking questions and respectfully listening, we give an experience that encourages him to become open and cooperative.

In short, since people trust their own experiences, we had better give positive ones if we wish to influence them.

# 13

## *Assume the Best of Others*

In human relations there is one attitude that continuously produces good fruit. It is the attitude of assuming good faith. This means to assume the best of others, to assume that they want to do well, that they mean to do well.

By acting on the assumption others are trying to do their best as they see it, though perhaps not as you see it, you can exert a powerful influence in bringing out the best in them. And vice versa.

Let me illustrate.

A friend of yours warns you not to trust your new boss. "He's cold, defensive, and simply doesn't care about his employees. I know—I used to work for him."

Accepting your friend's forewarning, you go forearmed. You keep up your own defenses. You guard your communication.

Your new employer senses your defensiveness and reacts similarly. He doesn't want to be hurt either. Seeing this defensiveness, what do you report to your friend?

"Thanks a lot, friend, I'm glad you told me. He was just like you said."

Now turn the illustration somewhat. This time you're the employer, and a trusted associate confides in you about one of your new employees—"a lazy clock watcher who'll produce only if you hover over him. I know—that's the only way I got anything out of him."

Grateful for the "inside" information, you hover.

However, the employee, with a concept of himself as being dependable and responsible, is eager to demonstrate his self-reliance and resourcefulness in this new job opportunity. His past job was only a means to an end. He wants new and challenging work with satisfactions within itself.

Now put these two attitudes together and watch what happens. "Sure enough," you report to your associate, "just as you said: the man's plain lazy, and hovering supervision's the only hope."

And the employee reports to his wife, "Let's keep looking around. There's no hope in this new job. I can barely wait till four-thirty every day."

These illustrations are typical of scores of daily commonplace occurrences in businesses, in schools, in neighborhoods, in homes. They are self-fulfilling prophecies. (Acting on a belief about the future helps to bring it about, thus self-fulfilling.)

In this very way the ideas and theories we have about leadership, management, parent-child relations, child development, or any subject where the human factor is dominant, tend to prove themselves true. We produce our own evidence. Attitudes create events.

Some, thinking themselves realistic, try to assume nothing; instead, they wait for the "facts" about people, to see what they'll do before making any judgments. These people also lose the tremendous power and motivating influence that is behind, first, clearly expressing belief and trust in others, and then, most important, acting accordingly.

Several studies in both the business world and education strongly point out the powerful influence of the leader's or teacher's attitude on the production and achievement of others. A classic one involved groups of low I.Q.-rated students. Most of the teachers were informed of the low I.Q. scores and taught accordingly. Some were not so informed, assumed normal I.Q. distribution, and treated the students accordingly. The unlabeled students consistently performed better than the labeled ones!

Our efforts to classify and categorize, judge and measure, often emerge from our own insecurities and frustrations in dealing with complex, changing, fluid realities. While our labels may appear neat and realistic and expedient, they may also be damaging, demoralizing, and highly unrealistic.

Each individual person is many things and has many dimensions, many potentials, some in evidence, most still dormant. He's a compound of many facts—even contradictory facts. He tends to react to how we treat him, what we believe about him.

Some may let us down. Some may take advantage of our trust, considering us naive or gullible. But most will come through, many simply because we believed they would. It is best not to bottleneck the many for fear of a few! Whenever we assume good faith, born of good motives and inner security, and then act accordingly, we appeal to whatever good there is in the other, even if there is very little.

The three wise monkeys put it this way: "Hear no evil—see no evil—speak no evil."

Goethe put it another way: "Treat a man as he is and he will remain as he is. Treat a man as he can and should be and he will become as he can and should be."

# 14

## *Empathy: A Problem Solver*

I'll never forget a teacher friend of mine who was heartsick over his relationship with his teenage son. "When I come into the room where he is reading or watching TV, he gets up and goes out—that's how bad the relationship is," he reported.

I encouraged him to try first to understand his son rather than to try first to get his son to understand him and his advice. He answered, "I already understand him. What he needs is to learn respect for his parents and to show appreciation for all we're trying to do for him."

For the son to really open up, his dad must work on the assumption he doesn't understand his son and perhaps never fully will but that he wants to and will try.

Eventually the father agreed to work on this assumption, for he felt he'd tried about everything else. I assured him he would have to prepare himself for the communication, for it would really test him, particularly his patience and self-control. He'd really have to have his mind made up.

The next evening at about 8:00 P.M. the father approached the son and said, "Son, I'm not happy with our relationship and I'd like to see what we can do to improve it. Perhaps I haven't taken the time to really understand you."

"Boy, I'll say you haven't! You've never understood me!" the son flashed back.

Inside the father burned, and it was about all he could do to keep from retorting, *Why, you ungrateful little whipper snapper! Don't you think I don't understand you! Why, I've gone through the mill. I know the story!*

But he restrained this impulse and said, "Well, son, perhaps I haven't, but I'd like to. Can you help me? For instance, take that blow-up we had last week over the car. Can you tell me how you saw it?"

The son, still angry and smarting inside, gave his defensive explanation. The father again restrained his tendency to rush in with his own self-justifying explanation but decided instead to continue to listen for understanding. He was glad he'd made his mind up to do this before the test came.

As he listened, something marvelous began to happen. His son started to soften. Soon he dropped his defenses and began to open up with some of his real problems and deeper feelings.

The father was so overwhelmed by what was happening between them—for the first time in years—and what he had wanted so badly for so long, he could hardly contain himself. He opened up also and shared some of the deep feelings and concerns as well as understandings he had regarding what had happened in the past. For the first time in years they weren't attacking and defending, but were genuinely trying to understand each other. What happiness it was for both!

Around 10:30 P.M. the mother came in and suggested it was bedtime. The father said they were communicating "for the first time" and wanted to continue.

They visited until after midnight and discussed many things, most of which were far more important to them both than the concerns they had been dueling and fencing around so long. The son had longed for a relationship with his dad, with whom he had identified when he was younger. Inside he had many self-doubts and mixed feelings he wanted to talk about. He would talk to his close friends about some of them but he found himself, in his desire to impress them, never being fully honest. Besides, they listened only in terms of their needs and experiences, so very little real empathy or satisfaction resulted.

The father told me of this experience a few days later and tearfully said, "I feel like I've found my son again and he's found his dad." He was truly grateful he had gone into the experience determined inside to first understand before trying to be understood.

It has always been impressive and instructive that the Prophet Joseph was so struck with the assurance that if he asked God for wisdom he would not be upbraided. Upbraiding means to accuse or reprove.

"I at length came to the determination to 'ask of God,' concluding that if he gave wisdom to them that lacked wisdom, and would give liberally, and not upbraid, I might venture."

Too often we punish honest, open expressions or questions. We upbraid, judge, belittle, embarrass. Others learn to cover up, to protect themselves, to not ask. The greatest single barrier to rich, honest family communication is the tendency to criticize and judge—in short, to upbraid. Watch closely and listen carefully and you'll find this tendency everywhere. Also notice what it does to you.

When we're communicating with another, we need to give full attention, to be "completely present," as one put it. Then we need to empathize—see it from the other's point of view, "walk in his moccasins" for awhile. This takes courage, and patience, and inner sources of security so we're not afraid of new learning or changing what we wanted to say before we began to listen.

# 15

## *How to Give an Understanding Response*

We've been discussing the power of understanding; now let's practice giving an understanding response. Here's the situation.

For several days you've sensed your fifteen-year-old daughter's unhappiness. You've asked about it but she claimed nothing was wrong, that "everything's okay." One night, while you're doing dishes together, she begins to open up.

"This rule that I can't date until I'm sixteen is embarrassing me to death. I like to follow our leaders' counsel, but all my friends are dating and that's all they can talk about. I feel as if I'm just out of it. Bill keeps asking me out and I keep having to tell him I'm not old enough. I just know he's going to ask me for the big beach party, and if I have to tell him no again, I just know he'll give up on me. So will Carol and Mary. Everyone's talking about it."

How do you respond?

First, think of what your most natural response would be. Would you say, "Oh, don't worry about it, honey, no one's going to give up on you," trying to give assurance? Or would you respond, "Just stick to your guns, Sue. Don't worry so much about what others say and think."

Neither of the above is an understanding response.

The first is an evaluative or judging response in terms of *your* values and *your* needs. The second is advice from *your* point of view or in terms of *your* needs.

Consider two more responses. First, "Tell me what they are saying about you." Second, "When they talk about you they are really secretly admiring you for your stand, and you're just feeling some normal insecurity."

Again, neither response shows that you understand Sue. The first is probing for information *you* feel is important. The second is interpreting what's happening with the friends and inside Sue, as *you* see it.

What would an understanding response be? First, it would attempt to reflect back what Sue feels and says so she would feel you, her mother, understand her feeling and her expression. Example: "You kind of feel torn inside, Sue. You want to follow what our leaders say but you also feel embarrassed when everyone else can date and you have to say no. Is that what you mean?"

She then may respond, "Yes, that's what I mean," and will go on, "but the thing I'm really afraid of is that I won't know how to act around boys when I do start dating. Everyone else is learning and I'm not."

Again, an understanding response would reflect back: "You feel somewhat scared that when the time comes you won't know what to do."

She may say yes and go on further and deeper into her feelings, or she may say, "Well, that's not exactly what I mean. I mean . . ." and she goes on to try to give you a clearer picture of what she's feeling and facing.

By using the understanding response (reflecting back her feeling), three things are beginning to happen.

First, both of you are really getting more understanding, you of her and she of herself. Because you weren't harsh ("Well, I don't care what they say, you know what the rule is!"), because you didn't rush in with judgment or advice or interpretation, thus taking direction of the communication from *your* point of view, she continued to open up into even deeper and more important problems.

Second, from increased understanding and clarity of the problems and feelings come courage and growth in responsible independence.

Sue didn't blame her mother or the leaders or ask for a change in the rule. All she expressed were some of the problems she was facing and her mixed feelings associated with them. If she can express them fully without fear of censure, embarrassment, or ridicule ("and upbraideth not"), she will become inwardly capable and desirous of coping with the situation herself.

Third, through such an effort to understand Sue, her mother is building a real confidence relationship that will prove to be immensely helpful to both over the next several years of schooling, romancing, courting, and marriage, with all the real temptations to stray that the world will provide.

Does all this mean that advice and counsel have no place and that the understanding response is the cure-all? Definitely not. It all depends on the situation and the people involved.

I believe the understanding approach has its greatest value when another person, particularly your husband, wife, or child, wants to talk about a problem or some feelings, when a lot of emotion is involved. If you seek to understand until the other feels understood and so states, it might then be most appropriate, based on your discernment, to give counsel, even strong counsel. Feeling understood and accepted, the other person will receive and respect your counsel better than before.

Test the value of an understanding response for yourself in three ways: (1) practice empathy when listening to another; (2) practice refraining from advising, judging, sympathizing, or interpreting; (3) practice reflecting or mirroring back the content, and particularly the feeling, of the other's expression.

In your practicing you will learn many things about others and about yourself.

One last word: the understanding response is more an attitude than a technique. It will fail if you're just trying to manipulate or figure out or psychoanalyze another. It will work if you really and deeply want to understand.

# 16

## *If Offended, Take the Initiative*

At the end of a speech on the importance of "going to the one who offended you," an individual approached me and said, "I liked your speech enough to do what you said. You offended me once and, frankly, I've discounted all you've said since."

He said that he was attending a fireside speech and had to leave for a minute in the middle. "As I walked down the aisle you commented, 'Don't run away mad,' and everybody laughed. I was embarrassed to leave as it was, but that comment, and everyone's laugh, knifed right into me. When I returned I sat in the back, still smarting and angry inside. I was so upset I could hardly listen to what you said then, and I felt about the same way even tonight."

This individual took the initiative to come to me rather than nursing his hurt and judging privately, thus fortifying the barrier between us. We both learned and benefited from the experience.

"And if thy brother or sister offend thee, thou shalt take him or her between him or her and thee alone; and if he or she confess thou shalt be reconciled." (D&C 42:88.)

Why is the initiative with the one who has been offended, when the natural tendency when we are offended is to say within ourselves, "He is the one at fault; therefore he should come to me."

Oftentimes a person offends unknowingly, as I had in the above situation. If someone offends you unknowingly and continues to do so, you are responsible for the strain in the relationship if you do not take the initiative to clear it up. Often you'll find you made unrealistic expectations. You may discover you simply didn't understand the situation at all.

One lady told me that for a long time she felt that her own husband had been unjustly treated by a leader in her stake. The resentment grew and grew until her children were similarly inflicted by this poisonous venom and the attitude of the entire family toward this man, his family, his business, and his stake leadership became critical and negative.

Eventually she took the initiative to go to him, and she returned with feelings of gratitude and sorrow—gratitude for clearing it up and sorrow because she learned the other side of the story. She had not acted on the entire picture. She was sick to think how long she had mothered such hostile feelings on the basis of a completely inaccurate understanding.

Consider two tragic consequences of not taking the initiative. First, the one offended often broods about the offense until the situation is blown all out of proportion. Like a poison, bitterness and resentment spread and afflict other relationships and situations totally removed from the initial one. Then guilt grows within, causing anger to flash and bite, feeding on the weaknesses of others. Eventually the mounting vindictive spirit can contain itself no longer, and it explodes irrationally at the slightest provocation on its "enemy," inflicting wounds and scars that may never be healed. Now the whole problem has changed, both in location and in complexity. The offended becomes the offender.

Second, sometimes we make expectations of another, and when he doesn't come through, we are offended. We then judge and behave defensively to avoid further hurt. The other sees this defensiveness and may react similarly, thus giving us new evidence to support our earlier judgments. We, the offended, bring about the very treatment we feared. This is the self-fulfilling prophecy.

Obviously, therefore, it's better not to take offense, whether intended or not. It's best not to judge another at all but to forgive "seven times seventy," if need be.

But if we are offended and we can't fully forgive or resolve it inside, we should go to the other shortly after the offense so reconciliation can take place.

I give two suggestions in taking the initiative.

First, we should do this in a good spirit, in control, not in the spirit of vindication and anger, to avoid giving offense ourself, thus compounding the problem. The roots of the courage to admit we were offended are spiritual.

Second, we should describe our feelings—when the offense took place—rather than judge or label the other. To say "I felt belittled and so embarrassed" is more accurate and less offensive than to say "your dominating attitude" or "your childish behavior." This preserves the dignity and self-respect of the other, who then can respond and learn without feeling threatened.

We must be aware that our feelings, opinions, and perceptions are not facts. To act on that awareness takes thought control and fosters humility.

# 17

## *Paying the Uttermost Farthing*

"My biggest worry and concern is my poor relationship with my fourteen-year-old son. I have set a poor example in the past with my yelling and losing my temper. How can I erase this image he has of me?" a father asked.

Perhaps there is no greater heartbreak than for parents to feel they are losing or have lost contact and influence with a son or daughter who is being drawn more and more into the lower roads of life.

What can be done in such a tragic situation? Fortunately a great deal can be done. Few, if any, situations are hopeless. There are yet several approaches, including the prayer of faith, which can be taken to heal the broken relationship and to exercise righteous influence again.

One of these approaches is to pay "the uttermost farthing." Consider very carefully a possible meaning of a teaching in the Savior's Sermon on the Mount:

"Agree with thine adversary quickly, whiles thou art in the way with him; lest at any time the adversary deliver thee to the judge, and the judge deliver thee to the officer, and thou be cast into prison.

"Verily I say unto thee, Thou shalt by no means come out thence, till thou has paid the uttermost farthing." (Matt 5:25-26.)

Applying this teaching to any seriously broken or

strained relationship—not just the family—I emphasize six points.

1.  We may honestly admit to ourselves, as the father above did, that we are at least partly to blame for the problem. Reflecting back, we can remember how we might have embarrassed, insulted, or belittled, or how we simply didn't take the time to understand, or how we were inconsistent in discipline or conditional in love. We may have felt justified at the time but now we realize that we simply lost control and gratified our pride. In short, we were unfair. We hurt another.

2.  When one is deeply hurt or embarrassed, he draws back and closes up. One of the safest ways to avoid future hurt from us is to simply distrust us. In this sense we have been judged as unkind, unfair, or not understanding, and put behind prison bars and walls in his own mind. Expecting nothing, he can then never be disappointed. He simply refuses to believe, to open up, to "release" us from the image or mental prison he has us in.

3.  Improving our behavior alone won't release us from this prison, simply because he can't afford to trust us again. It's too risky. He's suspicious of this new behavior, this new kind face, this "insincere" entreaty. "I trusted him before and look what happened."

Although inside he is crying out for parental direction and emotional support—playing roles and pretending adequacy is fatiguing—still we remain "judged" in his mental prison for an indeterminate sentence.

4.  Often the only way out is to go to him and admit our mistakes, apologize, and ask forgiveness. In this reconciliation we must become very, very specific in describing exactly what we did that was wrong. We must make no excuses or apologies, explanations or defenses. But let it clearly stand that we know we did wrong and that we are sincerely sorry. Then, in his own mind—where we are in prison—he knows we understand exactly what put us there and are paying the specific price of release.

Sometimes we make a stab at this process but inwardly

hold back, saying to ourself, "He should be sorry also. I can only go so far but no further until he acknowledges his part and seeks forgiveness also." This kind of peace-making is superficial, insincere, and manipulative. While it might temporarily calm the waters on the surface, the suspicious turbulence underneath still rages and the next stress situation on the relationship will reveal it. The "uttermost farthing" means exactly that. The uttermost—not the first, second, or third, but the uttermost.

5. This approach must be utterly sincere and not used as a manipulative technique to bring the other around.

If this approach is used only because it works, it will boomerang, for unless a real and sincere change takes place deep within us, sooner or later we'll trespass again on tender feelings and the new mental prison will have thicker walls than ever. He simply will not believe us when we say again how sorry we are. Repeated token repentance wins no confidence, human or divine.

6. I believe this approach will work in most situations, in time, both in obtaining a release from "prison," with its new opportunity to communicate and to influence, and in inspiring, not forcing, the other to make some hard admissions and resolves also.

# 18

## *Let Quarrels Fly Out Open Windows*

On December 1, 1969, a great storm, centered around the Aleutian Islands, spawned and drove huge waves toward the island chain of Hawaii, almost two thousand miles away. The surf built and built until some of the highest waves (50 to 60 feet) ever reported in Oahu's recent past began to pound her north shore.

It seemed so ironical: beautiful clear days, almost idyllic; yet the presence of this snarling, snapping, white-fanged sea monster.

The irony invited thousands of natives and tourists to come and see. But how deceiving! We thought we were in a good safe position, standing with everybody else many feet from the high-water mark of past waves, and then out on the horizon we could see an unusually large one rolling in. Everyone commented curiously at first, but as it came closer the danger became apparent and we ran. Twice that afternoon, hundreds of us watching from the so-called secure high shelf were enveloped in water to our knees.

Those who lived there were enveloped by terror. One couple watched in horror as a wave pushed their two-year-old girl, crib and all, out into the yard, where a wall then collapsed on her.

Many were literally sucked out of their cars; others were dragged off streets and out of service stations. A few were killed, many were injured, many were rescued. Scores of shore homes were blown apart; hundreds were damaged.

Days after the surf serpent had spent her fury we visited the destruction. I'll never forget seeing two homes, side by side, high up on Sunset Beach. One solidly built on a cement foundation was of good brick construction. The other was flimsy and frame, but standing three feet high on stilts.

When the waves reached the solid front wall of the first home, they had no place to go but through it. It literally exploded; all that was left was the good solid foundation and part of the side walls.

But when the waves slammed against the flimsy neighbor, they had somewhere to go—under it! It "withstood the rude blast" with almost no damage.

This whole experience reminded me of the German expression, "Let arguments fly out open windows." As I understand it, this means to give no answer to a contentious argument or an irresponsible accusation. Let such "fly out open windows" until they spend themselves. If you try to answer or reason back, you only serve to gratify and ignite the pent-up hostility and anger within, just as the solid wall ignited the pent-up power of the wave that destroyed it.

Your reasoning in such an argument may be sound, your logic consistent and convincing—but it isn't a matter of reason and logic. The battlefield is emotion, sometimes unbridled explosive emotion, and sometimes raw feeling veiled by a thin veneer of seeming reasonableness and sincerity.

As with the north shore that beautiful day, it may also seem at first a pleasant sunny situation, but the real source of the interpersonal storm that seems to erupt at the slightest provocation has its source in other places, in other problems, generally personal, and may have been building for days, months, even years.

When you remain silent, giving no answer, and go quietly about your business, the other has to struggle with the natural consequences of irresponsible expression. He or she may grow reasonable and may even apologize for taking it out on you or for being so irresponsible and childish. Sometimes merely restating or mirroring back the other's hostile comments will reveal to him his irresponsibility. But an answer only justifies the irresponsible spirit, and the argument reduces itself to an ego battle, however well masked by clever language. And no one ever wins one of these.

We must not allow ourselves to be drawn, either through our curiosity or our defensiveness, into any poisonous, contentious orbit or we will find ourselves bitten and afflicted similarly. Then others' weaknesses will become our own, and all this will sow a seedbed of future misunderstandings, accusations, and wranglings.

It is highly significant that the very first message the Savior delivered to the Nephites contained strong counsel against both doctrinal disputations and the spirit of contention.

"For verily, verily I say unto you, he that hath the spirit of contention is not of me, but is of the devil, who is the father of contention, and he stirreth up the hearts of men to contend with anger, one with another.

"Behold, this is not my doctrine, to stir up the hearts of men with anger, one against another; but this is my doctrine, that such things should be done away." (3 Nephi 11:29-30.)

The power to be still, to be patient, and to let arguments fly out open windows comes partially from understanding this very principle, but primarily it flows out of an inward peace and unity that is freed of the compulsive need to answer and justify. And the source of this peace is living responsibly, in control, and obedient to conscience.

# III

# FAMILY

# 19

## *Build Harmony in Your Family*

The late secretary-general of the United Nations, Dag Hammarskjold, once made this profound observation: "It is more noble to give yourself completely to one individual than to labor diligently for the salvation of the masses."

A father could be terribly involved and dedicated to his work, to church and community projects, and to many people's lives, yet not have a deep, meaningful relationship with his own wife. It would certainly take more nobility of character, more humility, more patience and understanding for him to develop such a relationship with one person, his wife, than it would take to give continued dedicated service to the many.

A bishop, a priesthood leader, or an auxiliary executive can be ever so devoted to working for the salvation of others, but perhaps be unwilling to do that which is necessary to build a rich relationship and meaningful two-way communication with a teenage son or daughter. To the many he serves by giving his time and talents, but to the one he may need to give more of himself, perhaps even his pride.

Some may even justify neglecting the one to take care of the many, feeling sustained in this attitude by many expressions of esteem and gratitude. Yet in quiet moments, within, we know differently. "No other success can compensate for failure in the home." (David O. McKay.)

9. *The habit of taking time with your key people —understanding, delegating, committing, training, encouraging, appreciating.*

10. *The courage to say no to the unimportant.*

# 30

## Keys to Effective Delegation

Delegation is the key to multiplying oneself. We delegate, of course, out of necessity: we simply have more work to do than we can do alone.

Let's examine the classic case of Moses and Jethro. Moses was killing himself off, trying to do everything for the children of Israel, to judge all matters, large and small. His father-in-law, Jethro, saw all this and advised, "The thing that thou doest is not good. Thou wilt surely wear away, both thou, and this people that is with thee: for this thing is too heavy for thee; thou art not able to perform it thyself alone."

Jethro then counseled Moses to do two things. First, Moses was to teach the people principles that embodied his judgments so they wouldn't have to come to him to decide every matter. They could reflect on the principles and think their problems through on their own. This is a powerful form of delegation—teaching true principles and trusting the people to apply them.

Second, Moses was to choose faithful followers and delegate all small matters to them, retaining to himself only matters of major importance.

Both of Jethro's recommendations required Moses to take more time at first in setting things up and to take risks. Instead of rendering judgments directly, he had to carefully select and train judges and put his faith in them. They might do it differently than he would. They might make mistakes.

However, Moses realized Jethro's counsel was right. The greater risks were *not* delegating. He delegated. (Study Exodus 18.)

Consider two reasons for not delegating: time and risk.

## 1. *Time*

Delegation does take more time in the beginning, and many who feel they are now pushed to the hilt simply won't take this time to explain, to train, to commit. Take the housewife who reasoned why she was still doing household tasks her children or other help could do: "I can do the job faster than it takes me to explain it. Besides, I do it better." Soon she accumulates so many things to do she feels even less time to delegate—to explain and train.

By analogy, her reasoning reminds me of the time I was too frantic picking up all my precious papers, which were blowing around my office, to take the time to close the window.

I'm convinced that we parents do many time-consuming tasks around the home that our children can and should do. But the time and process of identifying these tasks and of effectively training and committing our children to do them becomes the obstacle.

The initial delegating time spent, in the long run, is our greatest time saver.

## 2. *Risk*

To work through others involves the risk of doing things differently and sometimes doing things wrong. Often the top man in an organization, who is unwilling to delegate more than routine matters, has faith primarily in his own judgment and way of doing things. "It has brought me to where I am now. Why change? Why quarrel with success?" he reasons.

He has a point, and as long as he can continue successfully, we can't argue. Some people have extraordinary capacity and ability and can produce amazing results without delegating major responsibilities.

However, it somewhat depends on how we define success and results. Obviously people don't grow much as automatons, without solid responsibility for results and some freedom in method. In addition, organizations under such an arrangement are necessarily confined to the capacities of the top man. They reflect both his personal strength and weaknesses. To multiply oneself and to compensate for one's personal limitations require delegation.

The late J. C. Penney was quoted as saying that the wisest decision he ever made was to decide that he couldn't do it by himself any longer and that he had to let go. That decision, made long ago, enabled the development and growth of hundreds of stores and many thousands of individuals.

Many supervisors and organizations give lip service to the importance of delegation and development of people, but over a period of time, people learn otherwise. They learn to play it safe, to "make no waves." The politics of yesmanship and the art of mind-reading and second-guessing the boss are developed instead of resourcefulness and responsibleness.

Fearful of their boss and his autocratic, arbitrary ways, wanting everything done his way, they tell him what he likes to hear. Gradually, imperceptibly, he becomes insulated and isolated from what is really going on in the situation. His decisions and judgments suffer accordingly.

The boss didn't really want thinking, committed, responsible producers—he wanted carbon copies of himself. Consequently, the organization will perpetuate, not compensate for, his weaknesses and limitations. He also finds himself unable either to attract or to keep the very talented people he needs the most, unless they are rewarded in other ways.

In short, if we want responsible people and children, we must give them responsibility and hold them accountable. Consider the following simple four-step procedure in thinking through your own delegation opportunity:

1. Make a list of the tasks you do now.
2. Put them in the order of their importance.
3. Analyze each one. What is required to do it? Can it be delegated?
4. To whom? How? When?

Perhaps the crucial question is "If I delegate and trust another, am I willing to stick to my guns, to follow through?"

Delegation is the law of growth, both for organizations and for individuals. As with a child learning to walk, errors and mistakes are inevitably a part of the learning and growing process.

In the final analysis, effective delegation takes the emotional courage to allow, to one degree or another, others to make some mistakes on our own time, money, and good name. This courage consists of patience, self-control, faith in others and in their potential, and respect for individual differences.

# 31

## Three Steps of Effective Delegation

Effective delegation is very much like effective communication. It must be two-way. A responsibility is given. A responsibility is received.

There are three distinct, yet interrelated, phases or steps in effectively delegating responsibility.

### First, the initial agreement

This means both people have a clear understanding of what is expected and what resources, authority, latitude in method are given. This is the crucial step. It takes strong, clear thinking, a lot of two-way unguarded communication and commitment.

So far as practical, we should try to delegate by the results we expect of the person. Giving some freedom in method will help release the greatest potential in another. For when one is committed to results, he does what is necessary to achieve them. His creative potential is released. He'll grow the most with this approach, and so will the organization.

The typical delegating approach is to talk "duties" and "activities" and "time spent," which are methods in getting things done, not results.

The following are typical attitudes of people given responsibility for methods rather than results:

An employee: "I just knew it wouldn't work but he told me to do it that way. It's not my fault it didn't work out."

A daughter: "Mother won't like the way we do it anyway, so let's wait till she tells us what to do."

Whenever we delegate activities and specify all procedures, we retain responsibility for results ourselves. Perhaps this is the way we want it. That's fine, but let's not give the others the impression they're responsible for results or kid ourselves that we're effective motivators.

Rather, our attitude will likely become: "Unless I carefully follow through, I can't be certain the job will get done." Or we might even try to "hedge our bets": "Sometimes I even give two people the same job—unbeknown to each other—hoping at least one will come through."

When the expected results are obscure, neither person in the agreement knows how well things are going. Then, as with a vague legal contract, the likelihood of misunderstanding and personality conflicts are magnified many times.

Our real test in delegation comes when our employees or children do the job differently. If we think in terms of methods and procedures, to do things differently means to do things wrong. Then we can't bear to stand by and watch such mistakes, such neglect. So we step in.

When we step in and do the neglected work ourselves or have someone else do it; when we trounce someone for taking some initiative for doing it differently; when we double check everything and insist all decisions must be cleared; when we meticulously spell out every duty; when we overrule "their" decisions pertaining to "their" expected results; when we get rid of responsible yet independent thinkers and decision makers; when we multiply policies and procedures and rules—we take back responsibility.

And sometimes, in some situations, with some people, we should do this. But this is not delegating responsibility for results, and we'll need to provide closer, more time-consuming supervision to achieve them.

In short, we can't delegate results and supervise methods.

### Second, the process of sustaining the delegatees (employee, child, etc.)

The original agreement of giving and receiving a responsibility immediately turns the supervisor into a source of help rather than of judgment and fear. As one effective executive put it, "I choose good men, give them the job, and then get out of their way."

The supervisor becomes their helping advocate, not their feared adversary. He provides resources. He removes obstacles. He sustains actions and decisions. He gives a vision—the big picture—and provides counsel and training when sought. He shares feedback in the form of information about results just as soon as it comes in.

Whenever the person falls down on the job, on the original agreement, this supervisor's attitude is "How can I help?" rather than "What's wrong with you?" It may be necessary to reaffirm the original agreement or to make out a new one.

Then who supervises? we ask. The delegatee is supervised by results, by actual performance. His conscience (sense of responsibility, commitment, and integrity) is enthroned, not his boss. And it is always with him. Generally a man who has a clear picture of exactly what's expected knows in his heart how he's doing better than his supervisor. This is one of the reasons, when vision and opportunity are given, why people set high goals for themselves and are more strict in evaluating their own work than others would dare be.

### Third, the accountability process

The "days of judgment" are based on the original agreement or contract. It is largely one of self-evaluation, since result information was given as soon as it was available. This is also an ideal time to revise objectives and plans in terms of the current situation to challenge, to commit, to inspire, to appreciate.

There is no need to "fire" people with this delegation process. People are dignified throughout and will resign themselves or seek a new assignment, training, or special help to make them equal to their present one.

In contrast to the traditional approach, in which the supervisor evaluates and motivates, the follow-up process in this approach is always in terms of the original agreement. The delegatee evaluates and motivates himself. What time it saves! What human potential is released!

The key throughout this entire three-step process for the delegator—whether parent or supervisor—is to think clearly and to be strong and consistent within himself.

# 32

## *The Best Way to Learn Is by Doing*

The only way to learn how to play tennis is by playing it. Hearing about it, reading about it, watching others play it will help teach good theory, but good skill is developed only in practice.

This idea holds not only in the world of sports but also in less obvious areas of life, in developing true skill and competence in anything, whether it be how to give an understanding response, how to resolve conflict, or how to courageously confront another with certain realities.

Two principles of learning are involved. First, we learn *what* to do by listening, reading, watching, etc. Second, we learn *how* to do by doing, by practicing the *what*.

What to do and how to do it are two different kinds of knowledge and are frequently confused. Each kind of knowledge is vital and complements the other. One cannot be substituted for the other. Neither can one stand alone. For effectiveness, they depend upon each other.

What-to-do knowledge might be called intellectual or mind knowledge. How-to-do-it knowledge might be called instinctive, habit, or nerve-fiber knowledge.

Let me illustrate.

A mission president determined to teach the district and branch presidents how to give a call. He believed that if the calls were given correctly, resulting in a deep commitment, a fundamental cause of many problems would be eliminated.

The training meeting dealt with the great importance of giving a call right and with fundamental principles in doing so.

What happened? Some momentary inspiration and resolution. But shortly the leaders dropped back to their old ways and habits.

The leader then decided the district and branch presidents needed a second session to "see" the principles demonstrated.

Result? Again very little, if any, change. He wrongly assumed learning plus seeing would do the trick. He had again taught the "what" but not the "how." They were reconvinced but not converted, not changed. How to give a call is a skill, like tennis, and is learned best by doing.

Thus, the third training session provided opportunity for each person to practice giving calls, utilizing where appropriate the principles. They practiced all day—giving several calls, to different people, in differing circumstances. After each practice they'd get feedback from both an observer and the one receiving the call. Then they'd practice again. Then more feedback and theory. Then more practice in light of it. Then reflect. Then practice.

Something very basic was beginning to happen. Knowledge was becoming skill and their success thrilled them. They left that day fatigued but converted and happy. The effect in the mission was immediate in most areas. The leaders enthusiastically reported the results of giving calls right, both on themselves and with their people. Success bred more success.

Consider two additional implications for all of us who are interested in improving our own human skills and in helping others improve theirs.

First, learning by doing, however vital, is difficult. It obviously seems less efficient than telling or showing. It takes more time, more patience, more courage.

It usually involves an awkward phase of unlearning for many adults. Like trying to learn the right tennis grip, after years of doing it wrong, you don't know where you are for a while. It's uncomfortable. Sometimes it's downright embarrassing.

Second, when possible, it's best to practice in an environment that makes it easy and rewarding to learn from mistakes. You wouldn't practice your new tennis grip for the first time in a tournament.

I find most people are in this very dilemma in life: they know what to do but not how to do it. And they're afraid to go through the inevitably awkward mistake-making process of learning *how* for fear of embarrassment or ridicule. The guilt resulting from this "knowledge gap" is often crippling—unnecessarily.

A gentle home is an ideal place to learn human skills. Husbands and wives can even role play with each other how to communicate with their children on sensitive issues. The priceless skill of empathy is thus sharpened. Leaders and teachers can also design training programs that include opportunity for practice and for feedback.

When you think deeply about it, from an eternal perspective the principle of learning by doing is the essence of our purpose in mortality.

# 33

*Integrity:*
*The Foundation of Leadership*

A great deal is heard nowadays of the credibility gap. It's another way of saying: "Are they giving us the straight scoop?" "Can we trust them?"

These questions are felt, if not asked, everywhere—children ask of their parents, employees of their bosses, church workers of their leaders.

All of this inward doubting and questioning underscores the most fundamental but often neglected (with so much emphasis on technique, knowledge, style) principle of successful leadership: that the character or integrity of the leader is supreme.

The Lord gives a magnificent illustration of this as he contrasts three different leadership and teaching types or methods. Study the chart below in relation to John 10:1-15.

First note that since the shepherd (No. 1) truly cares for the sheep, he can be open and honest in communicating with them. He has no need to pretend or to manipulate from a distance. With pure motives, the sheep trust him and will also be open with him; thus, two-way communication. He has listened and understands their hopes and fears and needs. They know he cares, for he is kind and is willing to sacrifice himself for them. Therefore, he can lead them from in front through the drawing power of example and love. They give their loyalty, co-operation, and best effort. And their common goals are achieved.

But the hired sheepherder, a hireling (No. 2), has no such character. He's in it for his wage, whether it be money or power or even a better job, with more prestige. However, to win approval and to make good impressions, he pretends to care. Sometimes he professes his sincere intentions most vigorously. But since attitude communicates more eloquently than words, the sheep are puzzled. The trumpet isn't giving forth a certain sound. ("White man speaks with forked tongue.")

Consequently he can't lead in front. They won't follow. So he drives from behind and uses one approach after another to keep them moving or working. Carrot (reward) and stick (threats), hovering over, lecturing, "psyche up" cheerleading meetings, and other manipulations, such as buttering 'em up, chewing 'em out.

He doesn't need to wonder why attendance is low, why meetings and activities lack punch, why loyalty is superficial. "A double minded man is unstable in all his ways." (James 1:8.)

When the going really gets rough, when "the wolf" comes, his real motives surface. He deserts the sheep. He gives up on that ungrateful, rebellious son. He asks the bishop for a release or another job—and, of course, he has a "good" reason.

But sometimes he just resigns inside and grows indifferent and goes through the motions, like the sheep-type leader.

The sheep leader (No. 3) wants to be liked by everybody. He's often socially intelligent, knowing what others want, but has no vision or lifting power. He compromises the program, even the standards. His children and those he supervises like all the good and fun times—the course of least resistance—but when the going gets rough he can't understand why they desert him and follow a stronger-minded sheep.

Far and away the most important factor in leadership is the depth of sincere care in the leader. If we don't really care, all the latest techniques and leadership formulas will bring failure. But with it we can have success in spite of some bungling. As someone once put it, "I don't care how much you know until I know how much you care."

To become shepherds we must follow the True Shepherd.

## TYPE OF LEADERSHIP

|  | 1. Shepherd | 2. Hired Sheepherder (Hireling) | 3. Sheep |
|---|---|---|---|
| **Character Motive** | Love of sheep (people being supervised) | Love of wage ("What's in it for me?", glory, etc.) | Safety, security, belonging |
| **Communication** | Honest ("for they know his voice") Two-way: ("and am known of mine") | Dishonest, disguised ("know not the voice of strangers") One-way: his way or downward | Self-concerned, One-way |
| **Leadership** | Leads in front by example and love | Drive from behind— carrot (rewards) and stick (threats) approach. Hovering supervision | Follow—no vision, no drive, just go along like a "good guy" |
| **Consequences** | Safety, loyalty, self-realization, achievement of goals | Sheep deserted (resigns, is indifferent) when times get rough (when wolf approaches) | Course of least resistance; a Judas sheep could lead them astray |

# V

# GENERAL
# PRINCIPLES

# 34

## *Understanding Our Problems*

What are your problems?

A problem that can be understood is half solved. Consider three steps in understanding your problems.

First, think deeply about the problems that concern you most. What are they? Personal problems, such as a big career decision or the habit of procrastination? Family problems, such as improving your communication with your spouse or child? Financial problems, such as meeting payments or how to get ahead and save for college and missions?

Church problems, such as how to get people out to meeting, how to internally motivate the home teachers, how to get the priesthood leader to understand the needs of your auxiliary, how to release someone without offending them?

Work problems, such as how to get the ear of the boss, or how to secure more cooperation and dedication from your employees?

Or how to do all your church jobs without neglecting your family? How to handle rebellious teenagers? How to reach or reactivate an indifferent family member?

Second, classify all your problems under one of three categories: (1) direct control (own behavior, attitudes, decisions); (2) indirect control (others' behavior, attitudes, decisions); (3) no control (the past, natural laws and forces, certain fixed realities you live in).

This second step will take careful thinking and you may be amazed, if not chagrined, to find that you have no control whatever over many of your concerns and problems. Furthermore, you may have unwittingly acted on the assumption in the past that, in the name of position or authority or money, you could directly influence or control the behavior of others.

Perhaps you can buy a man's time, physical presence, or even his skill to do a particular job. You can almost force or pressure an employee or a young person to conform. But you cannot buy cooperation, you cannot buy loyalty, you cannot buy enthusiasm or initiative or resourcefulness. You cannot buy the dedication of heart, mind, and soul. You have to earn these things.

This is why some of us have been frustrated in the past; knowingly or unknowingly, we have assumed that indirect control problems were under our direct control.

Third, by using the same three categories, decide on a plan of action to deal with or solve the problems. In this process you'll discover one very simple, yet profound, truth. The answer to any of your problems lies in changing yourself.

Let me illustrate.

With regard to direct control problems—your own behavior—this truth is self-evident. If your problem is weight, you can immediately begin a regimen of dieting and/or exercise to solve it. If your problem is lack of ability to communicate, you can begin to take steps, such as acquire training, to overcome it. In short, direct control problems are solved by changing your habits of doing and thinking; in other words, self-control.

What about indirect control problems? You say, "Why must I change when it's my wife's (or husband's or child's or boss's) fault?" Simply because your past methods of influence haven't worked. If they had worked, you wouldn't have the problem, would you? Since they didn't work, you had better use new methods of influencing others. And this means you will have to change. You need to change your methods of influence, which means changing your own doing and thinking behavior. Again, self-control.

For instance, we all hear complaints from time to time that "if only the boss could understand my program or my problem. . . ." But few complainers take the time to prepare the kind of presentation that the boss would listen to and respect, in his language, with his problems in mind.

Now take the last category—no control problems. Since we can't control the problems, we can control our reaction to them. We decide within ourself how anything or anybody outside ourself will affect us. This attitude control frees one from circumstances and the judgments of others. We can learn from failures; develop patience and courage from trying situations; radiate cheer and hope in suffering. Our Lord is the supreme exemplar of this kind of overcoming, this self-control.

The great psychologist-philosopher William James put it: "The greatest single discovery of my generation is that we can change our circumstances by a mere change of our attitude."

We must look to ourselves for solutions.

"Keep thy heart with all diligence; for out of it are the issues of life." (Proverbs 4:23.)

# 35

## *Keep Means and Ends Straight*

It was going to be the best trip the family had ever taken—and the best vacation too. They were going east. A whole month's trip!

Oh, how thrilled the parents were, especially for their children! When they were young they had never had such a privilege. "Just think, kids," they would enthusiastically say, "to see the very birthplaces of our church and our country. When you visit the Sacred Grove and the Hill Cumorah you'll come to appreciate the truth and value of the Church just as we do."

At first the children were excited, but gradually, beginning with the teenagers, they grew indifferent and apathetic toward the trip and, at times, even resentful. They began to moan about having to leave their friends and all the summer fun on the social agenda.

The parents were both hurt and puzzled by this reaction. They had saved and prepared so long and held such high educational and spiritual expectations for such a trip! Now the children seemed so ungrateful, so unaware, so self-centered.

With the trip still weeks away, they were about to call the whole thing off when they discussed the situation with a friend who wasn't so emotionally involved.

This friend observed that the children might be reacting against the feeling that more value was being attached to the marvelous trip than was being given to them. "They may also be reacting against the fear of not being able to meet your high learning expectations."

A fear of failure, particularly of becoming unacceptable through it, destroys the very desire to try. Many people fear success for a similar reason: one success creates the expectation of more, which means more pressure and possible disappointment.

The friend suggested the parents stop pushing the trip and talking out *their* excitements and expectations. "Just live naturally and cheerfully, leave travel brochures and material about, and let the children express themselves as they naturally desire to. Don't judge their expressions; just listen to them. Listen to *their* interests, *their* enthusiasms, what *they* are looking to. Give value to your children rather than to the trip."

The parents did this and within a short time the children were all fired up about the trip. No one could talk about anything else, right up to departure time.

And the trip surpassed everybody's expectations!

This little family episode illustrates how easy it is to confuse means—methods and experiences—and ends, or ultimate purposes and values. These parents had placed more value on what they wanted their children to learn than on the children themselves. The children sensed this and rebelled by going in the very opposite direction, almost as if to test whether the parents put any value on them as they were. Once they felt assured of intrinsic worth and of their parents' unconditional love for them, they were freed of the need or desire to rebel. They were acceptable as they were and therefore could take on this new adventure without fear of becoming unacceptable if certain expectations were not realized.

But when we show respect only for certain *shoulds* of life and condition our love on conformity to these *shoulds,* we have a reactive, negative influence. Youth often then rebel against the very thing we're trying to teach under the popular, although defensive, banner "I gotta be me."

We have all seen people almost reactively driven into bad attitudes, bad experiences, even bad marriages, by well-intentioned but unwise parents who confuse ends and means by communicating conditional love and acceptance.

I saw this in myself just the other day in as small a thing as trying to teach my little son to swim. Placing more value on his swimming than on him—his level, interests, fears, and feelings—I found myself almost forcing through shame and comparison, through subtle threats and conditional love. Result? Hurt feelings and an aversion toward swimming in spite of my repentance.

The supreme value is the individual personality. Its growth and development according to the gospel plan is the supreme purpose. Everything else is a means to that end.

Outside of example—love's expression—nothing encourages a person to obey the sacred principles and laws of life more than our obedience to the laws of love toward that person.

## *We Reap Only What We Sow*

Hearing a knock at the door, I opened it and invited Clyde, a student of mine, in.

"I've come to find out how I'm doing in your class," he commented.

I had sensed a tendency to just get by in Clyde since the beginning of the term, and from other contacts we developed a good rapport together, so I felt safe in confronting him directly.

"Clyde, you really know how you're doing far better than I do. You didn't really come in to find out how you're doing but rather to find out how I thought you were doing, to see if you were 'beating the system.' You tell me, Clyde, just how are you doing?"

"Not very well," he answered. "I really haven't been able to put the time in I should have. I have such a heavy load and have been so busy with school activities."

I continued to confront him. "Clyde, aren't these just excuses for your own laziness in getting down to your studies as you should?"

He then opened up and admitted he'd been goofing off and that it was getting so late in the term he was beginning to worry and was now attempting to find out how he stood with each teacher so he could intelligently begin the cramming process.

The practice of "psyching out" the teacher, figuring out what he wants, how he tests, what one has to do and doesn't have to do, develops the attitudes of second guessing, masterminding, and appearing to be, as well as the skills of memorizing, regurgitating, and forgetting. As one student put it, "I don't work to learn. I just work to get good grades."

These tendencies are widespread not just with the youth in school today but with all age levels in all fields of endeavor. Consider your own past school experiences and habits, and you may find you too had these tendencies. I did.

The problem is that this approach in many social or manmade systems works. Some cramming experts learn to get by well in school without really learning how to think, to work, to communicate, to cooperate. Many whose personal and family lives are pockmarked with inconsideration, irresponsibility, and selfishness learn how to wear a different mask for the public and make quite an impression. They are successful for a while, but constant role playing is tortuous and fatiguing, and sooner or later a stress or dilemma situation will shear away their false facade, revealing the hypocrisy underneath. Justice is an exact taskmaster, and all accounts are eventually paid to him in full.

Even in church work we can strive for appearances of activity and faithfulness, so as to impress others, while inside we know we are not magnifying or being magnified.

Although its harvest in the long run is bitter, this shortcut approach is powerfully appealing, for it excuses consistent personal effort, initiative, and responsibility. Manmade religious doctrines of salvation are built upon it. Economic and political philosophies revolve around it.

I believe the key for parents, teachers, and leaders in resisting such shortcut doctrines and cramming practices is found in studying natural or God-made systems, as opposed to those that are social or manmade.

Take farming, for instance. Can you imagine a farmer cramming to bring in the harvest? You know, forgetting to plant in the spring, throwing some seed out in the summer, neglecting the weeding and watering, and then just before the big harvest really hitting it in an all-night session?

Can you imagine a mile runner, competing in the Olympics, cramming? Even though he looked great at the gun, within a lap the months of dissipation and violated training rules would show in his lungs and legs.

This means to raise your young with increasing amounts of real responsibility for results, where results can be seen, if possible. No escapes. No excuses. Appearances only are unacceptable.

This means to patiently teach and train them in the law of the harvest: we reap only what we sow. Then we must commit them, followed by showing trust in asking them to judge their own effort and performance, in terms of their consciences, their trained sense of responsibility. My experience convinces me that if we are honest and genuinely care, they will tell us how they are really doing and they will often ask for our help rather than pretending everything's okay.

This means we will also need to get close enough to them to do some honest confronting and to give candid feedback. We will need courage to keep from shielding them from the consequences of their actions and attitudes, particularly when some of those consequences might embarrass us.

Obviously to try to teach and do these things when we ourselves live by appearances, cramming, and shortcuts is like playing golf with a tennis racket.

# 37

## *Accept in Order to Improve*

One of the most common hangups people face in solving human problems is their own inability or unwillingness to face present realities. They refuse to start working on the situation as it is. They want it the way they want it or the way it should be.

To avoid facing and dealing with present facts is as foolish as a father saying to his son, "I don't care if the doctor says you've got rickets. You look perfectly healthy to me. Get up and do your work!" The very first step in that son's recovery is for both father and son to accept the fact that the boy has rickets! The next step is to begin to do something about it. But unless the first is taken, the next will never follow.

Take a wife, for instance, who constantly badgers and nags her husband to change. She refuses to accept him the way he is. "Of course I refuse!" she exclaims. "That's not how he should be! If I accept him, he'll never change."

However ironical it may seem, the first step in changing or improving another is to accept him as he is. Similarly, nothing reinforces present defensive behavior more than judgment or rejection.

Why is this so? First, simply because to be accepted is deeply satisfying and to be rejected is deeply threatening—like being eliminated from the human race. (One father actually told his asthmatic daughter to "leave the room if you have to breathe that way.") And second, because a feeling of acceptance and worth frees a person from the need to defend and helps release the natural growth tendency to improve.

Acceptance is not condoning a weakness or agreeing with an opinion. Rather, it is affirming the intrinsic worth of another through admitting or acknowledging that he does feel or think a particular way.

The apostle Peter, in substance, counseled, "Wives, if you have 'the word' and your husbands have not 'the word' and you want to bring your husbands to 'the word,' then do it without the use of 'the word.' Do it by your good behavior and by the unfailing loveliness of a meek and gentle spirit." (See 1 Peter 3.)

Many a wife or husband has seen miracles gradually happen in their homes once they stopped trying to reform their spouses and began to work upon themselves so as to be a light rather than a judge.

Look to your children for abundant evidence of the power of acceptance. Just recently I saw it in my six-year-old son as he learned to catch a baseball. At first he refused to play with the older children. He said he didn't care to play, that he wanted to do other things. The other things essentially amounted to spying on the others out of the corner of his eye. Actually, the problem was that he cared too much. The possible hurt and embarrassment of failure, of not being able to catch, outweighed the enjoyment of learning.

Then I saw my teenage daughter take him aside and let him know she accepted him and accepted the fact he didn't know how to catch very well but that she would teach him how to catch if he wanted her to. He did. Acceptance punctured the fear and sting of failure; in fact, it redefined it as a kind of success. Success is often on the far side of failure.

Consider three additional reasons why we often hold

back from accepting another or agreeing to begin working with the situation as it is.

First, it is so much easier to reject and judge than to accept and understand. It takes so little effort to preach the *shoulds* and so much patience and courage to deal with the knotty or the unpleasantness of what is.

Second, we think accepting certain realities is negative. To think positively is not to reject or deny certain seen realities but rather to accept them and then to believe in the unseen realities (the potential within), and to act accordingly. Our attitude can be "I accept you as you are but I treat you as you can and should be." For what a person is includes what he can become.

Few things are more negative and frustrating than that brand of positive thinking which denies the existence of things as they are and finds itself unable to give straight answers to simple questions.

Third, to accept another and to willingly and patiently work within the present situation, beginning at the present level, takes self-acceptance. This, in turn, emerges from honest self-communication and searching. This may be agonizing, for accepting another as he or she is now may make us feel responsible and guilty for the unhappy consequences of failure to do so in the past.

As it is put in boxing lingo, "You have to hit from where your fist is."

# 38

## *Mercy Must Not Rob Justice*

It was the night before the last day of finals. I could hear someone opening drawers and files in the office of another professor who I knew was out of town. A student shortly came out and explained to me he was turning in some late papers and had found the door unlocked.

After some checking about I was convinced this student had stolen the final exam, but the nature of the evidence was such that I would have to involve the other professor to clearly establish proof. I hesitated to do this, for I knew the teacher would immediately flunk the student. There would be no mercy. The student needed the class for graduation, which was to take place the next day. The student's parents and family had traveled a considerable distance to participate in all the final festivities and to see him graduate. He had his job lined up and was to start within a month. He was a very prominent school officer. On and on I reasoned with myself.

I decided to confront him directly rather than involve his professor. He denied everything and explained away all the circumstantial evidence I presented.

Again I debated within myself, finally deciding to let him know that I knew he had cheated but would not involve his professor because I felt the consequences on so many people would exceed his terrible wrong.

Almost a year later I asked an officer of the company he hired with how he was getting along.

"He's now with another company," was the answer.

"Why, what happened?" I inquired.

After pressing a little more, this company official said, "We have enough on him to send him to the federal penitentiary for five years." And then he gave the history: how outstanding his first months were—so outstanding they took a deep look and found all kinds of wheeling and dealing, some illegal, much borderline.

"Why didn't you confront him with the law?" I asked.

"We were afraid of the consequences. His parents, family—so many were involved."

How those words pierced my conscience! I wondered how much guilt was mine for letting "mercy rob justice." In fact, I found that this individual had a consistent pattern of getting away with things for years. He was able to talk himself out of almost everything. There was always an escape. A smooth talker, popular with many, trusted by none. Several of us, through his formative years, could see this pattern evolving and could have done something about it, could have faced him up to the real consequences of his own actions.

The cancerous spirit of lawlessness afflicting our nation today also had small beginnings. We can do something about the seeds we sow and how we tend them, but nothing about the harvest we reap. We have no control over consequences, only over actions and attitudes.

One of the kindest things, therefore, we can do for our children is to let the natural or logical consequences of their own actions teach them responsible behavior, justice. They may not like it or us, but popularity is a fickle standard by which to measure character development. Only sincere repentance, not mercy, can satisfy the demands of justice. (Study Alma 42.)

Insisting on justice demands more true love, not less. We care enough for their growth and security to suffer their displeasure. It is at this time, or shortly after their negative emotions spend themselves, that we need to "show forth an increase of love." They learn that law governs life and that we ourselves can be depended upon to be faithful to that law.

Whenever we, as parents or teachers or leaders, see a pattern of lawlessness or phoniness developing in our young people, then is the time to do some serious one-to-one teaching. Often, however, talking isn't enough; it may be *their* long suit. We need to clearly point out exactly what the consequences are if things continue. Then our consistent, kind-but-firm follow-through will eloquently communicate our sincerity and serious purpose.

Just as shock treatments help bring some highly disturbed people back to reality, so does candidly confronting someone we are responsible to, that we see through their phoniness, that we care enough for them to not let them get by with it anymore, and that we believe in them enough to expect more.

A life of pretense is so tortuous many literally hunger to be released from it by someone who they know "sees through me," who "understands me," and most importantly, who "cares enough to stay with me on the road back."

# 39

## *The Need for Meaningful Projects*

He was a restless boy. Irritable, too—always picking fights with younger brothers and sisters. He was uncooperative and bored. You could tell he was unhappy.

This teenager's parents were almost beside themselves trying to get him to change.

But through honest introspection and prayer, the parents eventually got a grip on themselves and refused to be controlled any longer by the spirit that he brought to the home. Then one day the father noticed, and was surprised by, his son's interest in some sketchy plans for a fence around the yard. He quickly seized the opportunity to involve his son. Little by little the boy became so involved in planning the project that he wanted to build it himself.

And build it he did. It took him several hours every day for over two months. He made a lot of mistakes—his father let him. But the final product was beautiful. And what a transformation in the attitude of the boy and in the spirit of the home! What a sense of achievement all around!

Just as soon as the teenage son found a meaningful project and reacted responsibly to it, all his energies were unified and focused. Reaping an inner sense of purpose and fulfillment, he lost the need to take his inner void and conflict out on others.

# THE BARBARY PIRATES

CHAPTER 1

# PIRATES OFF THE COAST
# OF NORTH AFRICA!

FOR CENTURIES THE BARBARY PIRATES HAD plagued the world. Long before any settler had set foot in the New World they had begun their raids on merchant vessels.

Cervantes, who later was to write the story of Don Quixote, was a prisoner of the Barbary pirates a generation before Raleigh's colonists landed at Roanoke in 1587. More than a century later Defoe, writing about a popular hero of fiction, Robinson Crusoe, told about his capture by, and escape from, the rovers of Sallee in Morocco.

How did this nuisance begin? Why did the civilized world put up with it for so long?

It should be understood that the Barbary pirates were not pirates in the real sense of the word. They were the citizens of countries which were at war with other countries. They captured prizes and took prisoners just as any warring nation did. At first the Barbary pirates had a religious reason for their wars: they were Muslims and they considered it their duty to make war on the Christians. When the Muslims enslaved their prisoners they were not behaving any worse than their enemies did, for in those days there were no international treaties regarding the treatment of captives.

Later on, when other countries began to observe certain rules in these matters, the Barbary States followed their example to a certain extent. They solemnly declared war and made peace. They kept their prisoners at hard labor and sold them for ransom, but in that hard world of long ago, prisoners could nowhere expect kind treatment. The ransoms that the pirates demanded were like the war indemnities and tribute money demanded in treaties of peace by other countries.

The name *Barbary States* came from a term originally used by the Greeks. Two thousand years before, they had called all those who did not speak Greek "Barbarians." This name was used in an effort to imitate the strange speech of foreigners, and it came to be permanently applied to the people of North Africa, the Berbers.

The homelands of these people—the four North African countries of Morocco, Algiers, Tunis, and Tripoli—were known as the Barbary States. They were parts of the vast Ottoman Empire which at one time had threatened to conquer the whole world. Later, this empire fell to pieces of its own weight, largely because it had never been able to build any system of government except a simple tyranny.

The Ottoman conquest of North Africa had not been very successful. Local generals, governors, and religious leaders managed to set themselves up as independent. At the same time they posed as dutiful subjects of the central government at Constantinople. But their rulers did not have an easy life, even if they lived in the midst of great wealth and enjoyed unlimited power.

The Dey or Bey, Pasha or Emperor, whatever the local ruler called himself, lived only as long as he could remain more powerful than his rivals and enemies. The moment his grasp weakened he could expect to be strangled and to be succeeded by someone else eager to take his place. The truth was that a large part of the people were no more loyal to their rulers than their rulers were to Constantinople. They paid taxes only when the ruler was strong enough to compel them; and they were often hostile and independent under their own chiefs.

It was only in the walled towns, and along the coastal strip, and in the accessible valleys, that the Muslim rulers could enforce their will. The pirate cities were often shut off, with the sea on one side and an enemy countryside on the other. So the rulers living in these seaboard towns came to be dependent for their luxuries, and even for their necessaries, on what they could steal from the outside world. The sea was far more open to them than the mountains and deserts that hemmed them in at their backs. With the loot they could win at sea they could buy their food from neighboring tribes. The slaves they captured could build palaces and fortifications for them, and they were thereby saved from any necessity to do honest work.

So to sea they went, capturing poorly armed ships, and often raiding the Christian coasts to loot the villages. The shores of Italy and France, sometimes even Ireland and once or twice Denmark, saw the Barbary pirates landing to carry off plunder and slaves. They exercised a certain amount of care not to anger powerful nations who might fight back. Often the pirates were glad to accept money instead of plunder, and ransom for the slaves. Up to a point money was more useful to them than either. But only up to a point.

The pirates must have war. Otherwise, the world would soon cease to fear them. Furthermore, among Arab pirates it was considered the mark of a gentleman to go out fighting now and then. So the Deys and the Beys went on raiding peaceful commerce. They knew perfectly well that if they stopped, there would be shortages of necessary goods among their subjects. These people would quickly find a ruler who would promise to manage things better.

Naturally the civilized world did not accept all this looting and piracy without protest. Over and over again European countries sent armed forces to North Africa. Spain and Sicily and France all sent their fleets and sometimes their armies. One of Britain's best admirals, Blake, was sent by Cromwell in the seventeenth century with a fleet that bombarded Tunis and for a short time brought order to the Mediterranean. Repeatedly, the European powers seized portions of North Africa and held them for a time. This was one of the best ways to control the Barbary States, for any Christian foothold in North Africa broke the chain of coastwise navigation that was important to a country of few roads.

Portugal provides another example of the struggle

against the Barbary States. Before Columbus discovered America, Portugal conquered Tangier and held the city for two hundred years. But the further history of the occupation is unfortunately typical. Tangier had to be occupied by Portuguese soldiers to defend it from the attacks of the Moors. Danger was constant and fighting frequent, and the occupation was expensive in money and men, while the returns in terms of trade were poor. The Portuguese could not make the place pay any more than the Moors could without piracy.

In 1662 Portugal was glad to rid herself of the burden by giving Tangier to England as part of the dowry when Charles II married a Portuguese princess. England raised a regiment or two and took over the occupation— the remains of York Castle still stand in Tangier as a reminder of the presence of the duke who later became James II. But twenty years of continuous warfare and siege wore out English patience, and the Dutch wars sapped her strength. In 1684 the garrison was withdrawn and the place reverted to the Moors.

The constant wars in Europe played an important part in allowing the Barbary pirates to continue so long as an expensive nuisance. Countries fighting for their existences could never afford to waste any of their strength on expeditions to Africa. The periods of time between wars were too short to permit long-term action against the pirates, although numerous attempts were made.

These attempts nearly all ended in a bargain being struck, after long haggling. The more powerful the country that was bargaining, the better the terms that were obtained. If the pirates pushed their demands too high the other power would fight sooner than pay. In time the pirates became really skillful in adapting their demands to the situation. They knew just the right sum to ask so that peace would be a little more profitable than war for both sides.

There were certain countries with whom the Barbary States never made peace. At that time, Italy was broken up into numerous tiny states—the Pope ruled Central Italy; Tuscany, Sardinia, Sicily, and Venice were independent, but their governments were mostly feeble and corrupt. As their fleets and their armies were weak, the Barbary States had no fear of them, and preyed on their shipping for centuries.

The pirates also raided their Italian coasts, to give the pirate fleets and their crews practice in looting. This proved to be an important bargaining factor when it came to haggling with the other powers. Moreover, such activities gave the pirates with a taste for fighting a chance to take part in their favorite pastimes without much danger. The raids also gave the pirates a supply of slave labor more convenient than that from across the Sahara desert.

One other factor must be taken into consideration. This state of affairs had lasted for centuries. British merchant ships had been exposed to capture by the pirates ever since the first ones had ventured into the Mediterranean. When the kingdom of France extended its rule to the Mediterranean, the pirates were already there. When Spain and Portugal freed themselves from the Moorish yoke, the new Christian kingdoms found themselves at war with Barbary.

The European shipping owner was inclined to think of losses he suffered at the hands of pirates as something that must be endured, for he had never known anything else. The attacks by the pirates added to working expenses, but so did storms and contrary winds. It seemed useless to hope that any of these evils would come to an end.

Finally, the problem was not an easy one to solve. It was possible for the European powers to bring a temporary halt to the pirates' activities. But for the Barbary States to give up piracy would mean that they would have to change their whole way of life. This was something they could not even consider. Under threats they would promise to keep the peace—they would promise anything. But in time, their lack of money and necessary goods would force them to return to their old way of life.

At the end of the Napoleonic wars, Europe used bombardment and blockade to teach the pirates a lasting lesson. Their slaves were freed, their ships captured, and their fortifications knocked into rubble. The pirates were forced to give promises of good behavior, but they were soon driven by their necessities into piracy again. Finally, France occupied Algiers and then—as had never been possible before—conquered the country foot by foot and replaced barbarism with civilization.

# CHAPTER 2

# AMERICAN SHIPS CAPTURED

WHEN THE YOUNG AMERICAN REPUBLIC CAME into existence, the situation in the Mediterranean seemed as far from solution as ever. Yet American merchant captains wanted to do business there. Shipping was an industry of vast importance to the young country on the Atlantic seaboard, just as it had been in Colonial days. Both as carriers and as traders American ships could make big profits, thanks to the excellent American shipbuilding facilities and the sharp American business sense.

The Stars and Stripes had not come of age before they were to be seen on every one of the seven seas, and they had no sooner appeared than they ran into trouble. Only a year after America and England signed the peace of 1783, a Moroccan warship, cruising in the Atlantic, captured the American merchant brig *Betsey*. The Moroccan captain had never seen the strange flag before, and it was taken for granted that the Ottoman powers were at war with any Christian nation with whom a treaty of peace had not been signed.

In spite of this occurrence, Morocco was the least troublesome of all the Barbary States. Its Emperor was a member of a long established dynasty and so he was fairly certain of his position. He protected his throne with the aid of a powerful bodyguard of African slave-soldiers who were devoted to him, and he enforced his rule by cruel methods. So the Emperor did not have to defer to the wishes of his ship captains, nor did he go in fear of being strangled if he did not give them the opportunity of taking prizes at sea.

Besides, Morocco, unlike the other Barbary States, controlled a large part of the interior as well as the coast towns, thanks to her comparatively stable government and regular army. So there was a regular food supply. Morrocan farms produced so much that there was a small amount left over for export. There was also a good deal of trade by the caravan routes across the Sahara.

Morocco, in fact, was a trading nation, and the Emperor saw the possibility of extending trade by friendship with America. He was willing to make a treaty; and one was finally signed. Captain Erving and his crew and the *Betsey* had lain captive at Tangier no more than six months before they were released. In the old sailing ship days, that was not much worse than anything else a seaman might expect in the ordinary practice of his profession.

The whole cost of the treaty between Morocco and the United States was no more than ten thousand dollars. This was a relatively small amount, for diplomatic relations with even a Christian power always involved much giving of jeweled snuff boxes and much paying of fees to minor officials. At any rate, the Emperor of Morocco was able to boast that he was the first neutral to recognize the existence of the United States.

Our relations with the pirate state of Algiers were quite different. The Algerine corsairs were hungry for loot. During the recent war, ships had sailed in convoy and pickings had been meager. Immediately after the conclusion of peace, Spain had turned all the weight of her navy upon the Algerines. She had barred Algerine ships from going out into the Atlantic through the Straits of Gibraltar, and had generally acted with so much resolution that they had been glad to make peace.

But peace once more opened the Straits to the Algerines and in the summer of 1785 the *Maria* of Boston and the *Dauphin* of Philadelphia were captured and brought into Algiers. They were the ships of a new and not very important country, which would provide welcome plunder and could not be expected to hit back. Algiers rejoiced when the prizes were brought in—there was always a celebration on those occasions. Then the ships and cargoes were sold and the crews set to forced labor.

Christian slaves were always greatly desired because the Muslims did not like to hold other Muslims in slavery. The captives were forced to do the degrading work which was considered beneath the dignity of an Algerine pirate. Furthermore, to treat the Christians harshly and to feed and house them badly was satisfying to Muslim feelings, and had the advantage of prompting the prisoners to write letters home with moving descriptions of their sufferings. As a result of these letters, the captives' relations or friends or government would gladly pay heavy ransoms for them.

The prisoners wrote to the American consul at Cadiz (their nearest fellow citizen), to friends at Lisbon, and ended by petitioning Congress. Nevertheless, they stayed in prison, such of them as did not die of disease, for eleven years. For at this moment the young republic was groping about to find a form of government; it had neither money nor power.

America did what little she could under the handicaps that beset her. She appealed to her former allies, France and Spain, and by their protests they actually succeeded in having the prisoners in Algiers treated a little better. But it was hopeless to expect either country to do more, to find money or fleets for a country that would make no attempt to provide them for itself.

Jefferson proposed the formation of a league of the smaller powers to establish a fleet which would keep the Barbary Coast under constant blockade. Half a dozen governments were agreeable. But the suggestion came to an end when the United States had to admit that she had no money, no ships, and no men to contribute. The other countries came to the natural conclusion that America was trying to get them to do her work for her, and the league fell apart.

Portugal, as it happened, was playing an important part at this moment. She had chosen to go to war with Algiers rather than continue to pay tribute, and surprisingly enough, Portugal was able to make herself respected in the naval war that followed. She took over the blockade of the Straits of Gibraltar and made it impossible for the Algerine corsairs to enter the Atlantic. At last American shipping could sail that ocean in safety.

As for the Mediterranean itself, the ingenuity and skill

of the American merchant captains prevented further trouble for a time. The Dutch and the Portuguese and the Spaniards were protecting the ships of their own nations with their own ships of war. There was nothing to prevent an American ship from sailing with such convoys and getting protection for nothing. Moreover British ships carried passes, and those passes were an absolute protection, thanks to British naval strength and well-judged bribes. An American skipper who was worth his salt could forge a pass, or bring an old one up to date.

Thus, trade was able to continue without any more Americans being brought into the Algerian slave pens, and the question never became serious enough to compel action by the United States. This was unfortunate for the prisoners already in Algerine hands.

It would have been very little comfort for those prisoners to know what their government was doing for them. Now and then the American government was making an offer. Algiers demanded sixty thousand dollars ransom; America offered four thousand, and would have found it hard to raise even that sum. Jefferson and Adams reported that peace with all the four Barbary States might be purchased for a million dollars, but Congress would appropriate only eighty thousand, so the prisoners stayed in prison.

A final step was to approach one of the several religious orders in France that devoted themselves to the ransoming of Christians from the Barbary States and to request them to undertake the task that the government felt incapable of doing itself. The negotiations dragged on slowly, for bids and counter-bids had to be carried across the Atlantic by sailing ship. Another reason for slowness was that all details had to be kept secret. If it became known how much America was willing to pay to free her citizens the Algerines would raise their price to that limit. Then all American citizens captured in the future would have to be ransomed at the same figure.

At last a series of events broke the deadlock. America adopted the Constitution, which made it possible for her to deal with kidnappers and blackmailers as they ought to be dealt with. Then the French Revolution brought about the breakup of the religious orders in France.

Finally all Europe burst into war. British sea power kept the French merchant ships in their ports except for occasional blockade runners. England's merchant fleets and those of her allies were forced to sail in convoys for protection against French privateers which were far more numerous and dangerous than the corsairs of the Barbary pirates.

As always in war, neutral shipping began to make increased profits. Every warring country needed ships to carry troops and warlike stores, but the need to travel in convoys slowed down the merchant fleets' activities. As a result freight rates rose while the neutrals, unhampered by convoy, reaped the advantage. Neutral ships could make still more money if they were willing to risk capture while blockade-running and contraband-carrying. At the same time the countries that were at war felt a greatly increased need for the neutrals' raw materials and manufactured goods. With this golden market open to her, Portugal could not afford to waste any time fighting

Algiers. Instead she made it her business to buy a hasty peace.

Strangely enough, this unimportant event, a peace between Portugal and Algiers, had a part in bringing about the foundation of the United States Navy.

Heretofore, the Portuguese had prevented the Algerines from passing through the Straits of Gibraltar. Now, with peace, the Straits were once more opened and the Algerines swarmed into the Atlantic. They had been long penned in, first by the Spaniards and then by the Portuguese, and they needed booty and slaves. They knew that in the Atlantic they would find both in plenty; there they would find the ships of a country that had not a single man-of-war to avenge an insult or to offer a moment's protection to her citizens.

At the end of 1793 appalling news began to arrive in the United States. A dozen American ships had been captured, ships from Philadelphia and New York and Newburyport. The Algerines had poured on board them, chattering and shouting in their unknown tongue, their

Oriental robes flapping and their Oriental beards flying in the wind. Madly intent on personal plunder, they had fallen upon the unfortunate Americans and stripped them of all they had.

The reason was this: The pirates had to give an account of all captured ships, cargoes, and crews to the Dey, who claimed his percentage. But the personal possessions of the crews were the prize of the first-comers. Watches and sextants and money were of enormous value, but shirts, trousers and shoes were also precious to the penniless pirates from Algiers. The Americans had to yield everything, in utter submission, for a word of protest would be answered by a blow from a scimitar.

There was no chance of offering any resistance. The American ships, even if they carried a gun or two (few of them did), had crews of only ten or twenty men, while the heavily armed Algerines often had crews of as many as two hundred. Their ships of war were fast and agile. In any case they usually managed to get within close range of their victims by hoisting false colors. People aboard vessels which were attacked knew that if they tried to fight, or if any pirate were hurt, every man in the captured ship would have his throat cut.

There was nothing to do but submit and be taken back to Algiers. There the captives were flung into a filthy prison, given starvation rations and set to work at heavy labor, with the lash for the sick and the weak. There was nothing to do but submit, and to write letters home pleading for rescue or ransom.

When the news of the acts of piracy arrived, America was better prepared to act on it. Reports came in from the American minister to Portugal and the American consul at Lisbon, telling of the losses. The Portuguese government had been persuaded to send some of their warships out as convoy for American vessels, but this was a favor that could not be expected to last for long.

The American minister to Portugal, writing to the Secretary of State, expressed a blunt truth. "It appears absurd to trust to the fleets of Portugal to protect our trade." He went on to say, "If we mean to have a commerce we must have a naval force to defend it."

Even Captain Richard O'Brien, the commander of the

*Dauphin* who had been a prisoner in Algiers since 1785, wrote stoutly to say that only in strength lay safety. John Paul Jones could be quoted, too. He had, of course, been consulted years before, and just before his death he had advised that the United States should act alone and with a naval force.

The arguments gathered force as they were presented to Congress. But the citizens who were opposed to our building an army and navy were still powerful and quite sincere. They were men of learning and experience who believed that the creation of a regular armed force would endanger the freedom of the republic. They believed that an "officer caste" or a successful commander might one day take over the government of the United States. They believed, too, that because this danger existed, it would be better for the United States to go on enduring the enslavement of her citizens and the loss of her ships.

There was another section of the opposition—James Madison was its spokesman—who believed that the establishment of a navy might lead to difficulties with other naval powers. These men did not give enough thought to the difficulties that might arise in the absence of a navy.

The opposition was strong enough to force a change in the proposed law: If peace were to be made with Algiers, then the work on the ships authorized by the law was to stop. With that concession, the bill passed, and in March, 1794, the United States Navy was born. The President was given the power to start building six frigates. Congress was careful to prescribe what officers and men were to be employed, how they were to be fed, and how much they were to be paid.

Later on, Congress took the final step of appropriating two-thirds of a million dollars for the expenses of the navy. Thereupon the *United States,* the *Constellation,* the *Constitution,* and the other ships which were to make naval history came into being.

Time was to prove that Congress, with all its care, had not troubled to legislate on a most important matter. By not troubling, Congress made another great contribution to naval history. The lawmakers had neglected to name the person who was to design the vessels. The credit for the nomination must go to President Washington, and we first hear the great names of Joshua Humphreys and of his assistant, Josiah Fox.

All countries occasionally pass through periods when they produce a whole generation of great figures. During these periods, outstanding men and women appear in every human activity and add luster to the arts of peace as well as to the arts of war. The Elizabethan Age in England produced men of genius of all kinds, and so did the Revolutionary period in America. Franklin and Washington, Jefferson and Hamilton and Madison—there is no end to the list of men of superlative talent and character.

The name of Joshua Humphreys must be added to the list, as the outstanding designer of warships of his period. He had the clarity of vision that enabled him to decide exactly what type of ship would best serve the purpose of his country, and he had the technical skill and knowledge to carry out his ideas. It was almost equally important that he had the persuasive power and the personality that enabled him to induce other people to agree with him.

Humphreys built ships that were made to endure both battle and storm. He packed them full of fighting power, and he gave them the speed and maneuverability which enabled them to overtake the weak and escape from the strong. At a time when every country in the world was fighting for national existence and calling upon its naval designers to build better ships, it was Humphreys who came forward with the best designs. He produced the ships; it was for America to produce the men.

CHAPTER 3

# U.S. ATTEMPTS BLOCKADE
# OF TRIPOLI HARBOR

A VERY UNHAPPY CHAPTER IN AMERICAN history came gradually to a close. The period of uncertainty and doubt came to an end. At various times government leaders had decided to fight rather than pay blackmail to the Barbary States—but they had continued to pay the blackmail. They had decided, too, that it would be wrong to make payments in the form of naval stores, for the Barbary States would use these against American vessels—but they had sent the naval stores: weapons, ammunition, supplies, even ships.

They had even searched Europe for jeweled pistols

and daggers that might suit the taste of the African rulers. They had submitted more than once to having American merchant ships captured and American citizens enslaved. They had endured the crowning humiliation of seeing an American frigate obeying the orders of the Dey of Algiers to carry presents for him to Constantinople.

Now and then the government of the United States had taken action to avenge these injuries. However, the action lacked force because President Jefferson decided that he could not, under the Constitution, consider the United States to be at war with Tripoli, even though Tripoli was at war with the United States. The result of this was seen when the schooner *Enterprise* fell in with the Tripolitan ship of war *Tripoli,* outmaneuvered her, fought her, beat her into a wreck and forced her to surrender, and then allowed her to go free again.

The Constitution was young then, and it was every man's duty to be as careful about it as he could be. It was only six months later—in February, 1802—that Congress solved the problem by authorizing the President to take whatever action he thought necessary for the protection of the seamen and commerce of the United States.

It was then that an extra word appeared in the orders given by the Secretary of the Navy to the naval officers of the United States. They were ordered to "take, sink, burn, or otherwise destroy" the ships of the enemy. That very phrase had appeared for centuries in the orders given to officers of the British Navy. The extra word "take" made all the difference. Until then our naval officers were ordered only to sink, burn, and destroy, which was one more example of the difficulties that must arise in a badly defined international situation.

In 1801 Tripolitan captains could save their ships and themselves simply by surrendering. This strange situation existed, despite the fact that three months before the battle, the Pasha of Tripoli had declared war on the United States and had insulted the American flag. These events took place after the Pasha had had five years of peace. Almost his first act in 1796, when he succeeded his father (and murdered one brother and drove another out of the country), had been to make peace. Now he felt that he had not made nearly so profitable a bargain as had his neighbors of Morocco and Algiers and Tunis. He hoped war would be more profitable.

Already, in anticipation of trouble with the Pasha, the United States government had taken precautionary steps. A squadron of American ships had been ordered to the Mediterranean. Thus, the United States was brought face to face with a whole series of naval problems which demanded solution. The first one—where to get the necessary ships—was already solved, for vessels were available. Although the 1796 treaty of peace between the United States and Tripoli had been signed before the ships which Humphreys designed were completed, some of them were nearly finished. President Washington had then persuaded Congress to authorize completion, and the others were finished as a result of the brief war with France in 1798 and 1799.

Now, no one doubted that the small squadron which could be sent immediately was large enough to command the Mediterranean—that was the clearest proof of the weakness of the Barbary powers. Everyone knew that if the pirates contested the command of the sea in a pitched battle they would be beaten, which makes it stranger still that the world had tolerated this nuisance for so many centuries.

So there were enough ships; the next thing was to find officers to command them, and that was more difficult. The service was young, but several of the captains were already too old to endure the hardships of long service at sea. Furthermore, the Navy suffered a severe blow when Thomas Truxtun, who in the *Constellation* had so brilliantly captured the *Insurgente* in 1799, refused the command on a point of etiquette.

America had to hunt for a new commander of the Navy, and eventually employed five during the four years that the war lasted. That is not a surprising fact, for men fit for independent command are hard to find. The difficulties regarding the command in the Mediterranean came to the government's notice only as the war progressed. It appeared when the war began that Richard Dale, who as a very young man had been first lieutenant of Paul Jones's *Bonbomme Richard,* was quite suitable, and he became the first commander of the Navy. There were also many junior officers whose brilliance was guessed at if not already proved.

The officers could be found; it was a little harder to find the men. Most of them had to be trained seamen, for the sailing ship seaman was a highly skilled craftsman. Habitually when he went aloft to set sail or to shorten sail he performed feats which equaled those of circus performers. Often he had to perform those feats in the dark, high up in the rigging of a ship that rolled and pitched wildly in a rough sea. Often, too, every rope and piece of canvas that he laid hands on was covered with ice.

To steer a ship in good weather on a steady course so as to lose neither time nor distance was an art hard to learn. To do so in a storm with everyone's safety depending on quick and exact handling of the wheel called for years of experience.

The seaman was a man of a hundred skilled trades. Even making the best use of one's weight and strength in a team working a windlass or hauling on a rope was a knack that had to be acquired. A very brief training would make a man a gunner, but a man could not be called a seaman without at least a year at sea.

So to man the warships of the United States the seamen were necessary, and it was not easy to attract seamen into the service. With the wartime boom, merchant seamen were enjoying good wages and full employment. Consequently, they thought twice about giving up these advantages in exchange for the lower pay authorized by Congress and submitting themselves to the severe discipline of a ship of war and enduring the additional hardships of long months at sea.

There were patriotic men who enlisted for the one-year engagement that the Navy offered, but the numbers had to be filled up with whatever men came to hand. In this latter group were men who could not, for various reasons, find employment in merchant ships and foreign seamen whose usual wages and living conditions were even lower than those in the United States Navy. There were also landsmen who would have to be taught. Dale's instructions from the Secretary of the Navy included a hint that he could "accept the services" of any prisoners of war who might volunteer.

When the ships with their officers and men and stores were ready, it had to be decided how Dale was to use them. It would be foolish to sail such a fleet four thousand miles to Tripoli without a clear idea of what it was to do on arrival there. The Pasha had to be forced to agree to American terms; what was the best method of exerting force? Capturing Tripolitan ships would be effective, but the moment the alarm was given, every Tripolitan ship that could not get home would seek shelter in a neutral harbor. What next?

It might seem obvious that the next thing to do would be to enter the Tripolitans' harbor, capture the shipping there, and threaten to lay the whole place in ruins. But that was not so easy; the harbor was guarded by batteries and fortifications with scores of heavy guns. Wooden ships fighting stone walls were at a sad disadvantage.

The harbor, too, was shallow and difficult to enter, and the Tripolitans had a flotilla of gunboats. These were small craft that carried only one or two heavy guns, but those guns could send their shot even through the stout sides of the *President*. The gunboats were of shallow draft, and they could be moved about by oars, so that they could take shelter among shoals where the American frigates could not reach them. So bombardment of the town was likely to be dangerous and expensive and it might well fail. The orders to Dale did not contemplate bombardment.

The real weakness of Tripoli, which dictated the plan of campaign, was the dependence of the town on outside sources of supply. The roads into the town were bad, so foodstuffs were habitually brought in by sea. If no ships were allowed to enter, the town would have no more food than could be collected in the immediate neighborhood. It was hoped that starvation would soon bring the Tripolitans to their senses.

Grain and meat were imported into Tripoli from various points along the coast, from Italy and Spain, while fishing played an important part in the Tripolitan economy. At that time and for centuries before, the tunny fisheries on the Libyan coast were a productive industry as they are to this day. Bottling up the fishing fleets and cutting off the coasting trade should be effective.

And the Tripolitans depended on the sea for their luxuries as well as their necessities; blockade would keep the corsairs idle, and there would be no more gala days to celebrate the arrival of prizes. The pirate captains who had a voice in the government of the city would not like that, and if they grew restless the Pasha could fear dethronement and assassination.

So the orders to Dale directed him to sweep the enemy's ships from the sea and then to establish a blockade of Tripoli. He was to maintain the blockade until the enemy was willing to agree to terms of peace. Nobody believed that the blockade would be difficult to enforce, or that it would have to be long maintained. Thus it would be inexpensive—especially inexpensive in lives—and the United States government confidently expected that a cheap and easy victory would be won. A summer's campaign ought to humble the Tripolitans. No one stopped to wonder why, if it was as easy as that, the

Barbary pirates had managed to exist for centuries in the face of the hostility of the rest of the world.

There were special reasons which were not easy to appreciate at first. The principal one was geographical. The North African coast is difficult and dangerous. Shallows extend far out, and there are very few harbors. When the wind blew from the sea to the shore—as it did more often than not—a sailing ship was in grave danger of being forced aground. The danger was made greater still because there were no reliable charts and because the shore lay so low and was so featureless that it was hard to determine one's position. A north wind meant terrible danger, and a south wind was likely to blow the blockading ships away from their station.

The coasting and fishing vessels that supplied Tripoli with food were very small. They could creep along in the shallows out of reach of the big ships, and in a calm they would use their oars. By the aid of their local knowledge they could make their final run into the town at night, out of sight of the blockaders. Even a small flow of provisions into the town would make a big difference in the situation there. If only half the usual supply came in, and there were six months' provisions on hand, the town could endure a year of blockade. It could hold out far longer if the people made a sharp cut in their use of food and other necessities. And Dale's seamen were only enlisted for a year!

The other geographical difficulty arose from the distance between the Mediterranean and America. A ship did well if she arrived off Tripoli a month after leaving Hampton Roads. After Dale reached the Mediterranean, it took two months, and often longer, for him to receive a reply to any letter he wrote to his government. Every cannon ball he fired, every barrel of beef his men ate, had to be replaced from four thousand miles away. Sails and cordage wore out fast when continually at sea. If the *Constitution* were to split a topsail in a squall, Dale could count himself lucky if three months later he received a new one.

What Dale needed was an "advance base" somewhere close to Tripoli where stores could be accumulated, his ships refitted, and his men rested. But there was no place in Africa at all suitable, and if there had been it would have taken a military garrison to hold it secure.

There were plenty of friendly ports in the Mediter-ranean, and the European powers were friendly to Dale's squadron, but Europe was convulsed with war. The ports under British control were hard put to it to supply the British Navy. The ports under French control had been blockaded by the British for years and were experiencing the worst of wartime shortages. When most of the world was locked in desperate combat it could hardly be expected that anyone could spare help for the little American squadron.

For it was only a little squadron—the *President,* the *Philadelphia,* the *Essex,* and the *Enterprise,* a big frigate, two small ones, and a schooner. The squadron was big enough to command the Mediterranean and to scare every Tripolitan ship of war into harbor, but it was not big enough to conduct a war. There were only four ships. Suppose one was employed watching Algiers and Gibraltar, a second was convoying American merchant ships, and a third ran aground and damaged herself—as actually happened to the *Constitution*—how was the blockade to be conducted when the fourth ship ran short of water and had to go off for more? And how were messages to be sent? How was contact to be maintained with the other Mediterranean powers?

Those were problems which Dale had to try to solve, and they were also the problems which faced the American people and the American government. They had entered into a war, and, as happens ninety-nine times out of a hundred, they had underestimated the effort necessary to win it. It remained to be seen if they would have the resolution to see the business through.

# CHAPTER 4

# COMMODORE MORRIS FAILS TO SUBDUE PIRATES

EVEN THOUGH DALE EVENTUALLY DID BADLY with the forces under his command, he began astonishingly well. He came into Gibraltar in the nick of time after having spent a month crossing the Atlantic. Nelson once said, "Lose not an hour" and Dale's arrival was one more example of the importance of hours in naval warfare, for in Gibraltar he found two Tripolitan ships on the point of going out into the Atlantic to capture prizes.

These ships were under the command of the most formidable of the Tripolitan captains, a European who, taken prisoner by the Tripolitans years before, had changed his religion and his name. He was now called Murad the pirate instead of Peter Lisle the Scot, just as his flagship, which had once been the *Betsey* of Boston, was now the *Meshuda,* twenty-eight guns.

Had Dale been even a day later Murad would have been loose in the Atlantic and could have done very great damage. As it was, Dale came sailing in, saluted the British authorities in Gibraltar, anchored beside Murad, and announced his intention of fighting the pirate the moment he put his nose outside neutral waters. Murad said there was no war as yet (though two months before the Pasha of Tripoli had declared war and cut down the American consular flag), but Dale did not believe him. He left the *Philadelphia* to watch Murad while he himself went on with the rest of the squadron into the Mediterranean.

Murad with his two ships looked out at the *Philadelphia* and did not like what he saw. The British authorities, while they maintained the neutrality of the harbor, would not lift a finger to help him. His stores and water threatened to run short, he faced destruction outside the bay and ruin inside, and in the end abandoned his ships, leaving them in charge of a small maintenance party. He then scuttled across the Straits with his crews in the ships' boats. From Tetuan he and his men tried to get back to Tripoli, but Murad was one of the few who succeeded. For years after, his ships swung useless at their anchors in Gibraltar Bay. Thus, at least a third of the Tripolitan fleet was disposed of.

Dale went on up the Mediterranean, showed his formidable ships of war to Algiers and Tunis, making a very healthy impression, and then proceeded to Tripoli.

So here he was, at the enemy's gates, so to speak. What next? Tripoli was decidedly alarmed. The Tripolitan batteries were manned, the gunboats took shelter under their protection, and the coasting vessels hid themselves away.

Dale with only one ship, the *President,* had been able to make the pirates tremble. The *Philadelphia* he had left at Gibraltar; the *Essex* was on convoy duty. The schooner *Enterprise* began to run short of water and was sent off to Malta to fill up.

Alone, Dale waited for Tripoli to offer peace; Tripoli waited to see what would happen. For two and a half weeks the two sides looked at each other. Now the *President* was running short of water—it was five weeks since she had filled up at Gibraltar—and in Dale's opinion there was nothing else to do but to go to Malta himself to obtain more.

So it was that one morning the astonished Tripolitans looked out over the Mediterranean to find that the coast was clear. The big American frigate had gone. Horsemen took the news along the coast; soon provisions would once more enter Tripoli.

Not only that; the *President* had barely left when a battered ship came creeping into Tripoli under a single sail. She was the *Tripoli,* with thirty wounded on board, having thrown twenty dead overboard, her sides torn with shot and one mast missing. Lieutenant Andrew Sterrett, commanding the *Enterprise,* had encountered her on his way to Malta, and by the brilliant way in which he had handled his ship had utterly defeated her without losing a man himself. The Tripolitans heard the news about the fighting capacity of the Americans with some dismay. On the other hand, there was the astonishing fact that the Americans had set the ship free after capturing her. They had not looted the vessel, and they had not enslaved the crew.

The Tripolitans could hardly be expected to understand the Constitution of the United States or to appreciate Mr. Jefferson's regard for it. They could only reach the conclusion that the Americans knew nothing about waging war, and that they could look forward to wringing more blackmail from this unwarlike nation.

The Tripolitans did not worry at all when American ships showed up now and then to continue the blockade—whenever Dale had a ship available. And before a month was out they had a fresh example of the trusting innocence of these Americans.

Dale, returning from Malta, met a Greek ship heading for Tripoli. He turned her back, in accordance with the laws of blockade. (He could not make her a prize, as she could claim that the news of the blockade had not reached her.) But on board there were forty Tripolitan passengers, including an officer and twenty soldiers. Dale took them prisoners, and then actually landed them all in exchange for the Pasha's promise that he would give three Americans in exchange. There were no American prisoners in Tripoli at the time, and the Pasha's promise was worth no more than any pirate promise in any case.

There could be nothing more encouraging for the Tripolitans. An enemy who proclaimed a blockade and did not enforce it, who took prizes and then returned them, who took prisoners and then set them at liberty, was not an enemy to be feared. Presumably he was therefore an enemy who could be bullied into paying substantial blackmail. Was it not well known that America was sending to the other Barbary States a steady stream of presents—money, jewels and naval stores? The spirits of the Tripolitans rose steadily; so did their demands, and so did their determination to fight it out until those demands were satisfied.

The other Barbary States, who of course had been watching the contest with the deepest interest, began to grow restless. They began to think that they were not being paid enough by the United States. They grew more and more exacting in their demands. They objected to the small hindrance imposed on their trade by Dale's blockade of Tripoli. American consuls were treated with increasing insolence, and ships of war began to be fitted out in the ports of Morocco and Algiers and Tunis.

The unfortunate Dale, as if he had not already enough to worry him, was now alarmed by these menaces. His tiny force had been too small even to watch one single port in the Mediterranean; he could not hope to watch half a dozen more.

Another of his worries resulted from the quick passage of time. Many of his men in the *President* had begun their one year's enlistment as early as April, 1801. Now it was February, 1802, and at that time of year, with the westerly gales blowing, it might take two months or more for his ships to return to America from far inside the Mediterranean. The engagements the United States had entered into with her seamen must be honored.

So Dale sailed for home with his flagship, depriving his

squadron of their leader, and leaving his captains to quarrel with each other. They also quarreled with the United States consuls, who were not only trying to conduct negotiations but were also trying to press plans of campaign of their own devising upon them. It was a miserable end to Dale's command.

But Dale arrived in the United States to find America resolved not only to go on with the blockade, but to exert herself even more in the endeavor to find an honorable peace. More ships were being fitted out; a new commodore had been selected—Richard V. Morris—and no fewer than seven more frigates were destined for service in the Mediterranean. Dale's largest force had amounted to five frigates and a schooner; Morris would have twelve frigates and a schooner if every ship joined him. Surely with that force he could accomplish everything necessary in the Mediterranean, especially now that Congress had empowered the President to fight against America's declared enemies.

America was convinced, as she watched Morris sail away, that this new expedition would soon come home victorious. So profound was this conviction that the administration, suddenly alarmed about the cost of all this, decided that Morris's force was over-large, and recalled two of his frigates.

Morris sailed out from Norfolk in May, 1802, but with contrary winds did not succeed in getting clear of Hampton Roads for two days. He took just four weeks to cross the Atlantic, and arrived at Gibraltar with his ship, the *Chesapeake,* in need of refitting. It was fortunate that at this moment England was at peace with Napoleon, and so all the facilities of the dockyard at Gibraltar were put at Morris's disposal. Three weeks' hard work were required to get the *Chesapeake* ready for sea again and to replace her cracked mainmast, for the United States dockyards had not done their work well.

And while Morris waited at Gibraltar, one item of news reached him after another, each more harassing than the one before. Morocco was threatening trouble. Her Emperor wanted to resume trade with Tripoli, and he wanted to take possession of the *Meshuda*—once the

*Betsey* of Boston—which was still lying in Gibraltar Bay in charge of Tripolitan caretakers. Morris refused. There was no sense in blockading Tripoli and yet allowing Moroccan ships to enter, nor was there any sense in permitting an increase in the naval strength of a possible enemy.

Morocco was enraged at the refusals. She threatened war, and the American consul, who knew his duty was first to keep peace between Morocco and America, became alarmed and pelted Morris with protests.

That was not the end of Morris's trouble. There were numerous American ships inside or just outside the Mediterranean. It was Morris's business to provide convoy for them, but he simply did not have enough ships to do so and still watch Morocco. The American captains naturally refused to keep out of danger because they would thereby lose profits. So it was not long before news arrived that the *Franklin* of Philadelphia had been taken by a Tripolitan corsair which had slipped out of Tripoli and returned with four American prisoners.

Now Tripoli could apply still greater pressure upon

the United States. Of course no one in Tripoli paid any attention to the Pasha's old agreement with Dale over the twenty Tripolitan prisoners Dale had returned.

Other news came in—trouble and more trouble. Captain Alexander Murray in the *Constellation* had had a skirmish with the Tripolitan gunboats. He had found them close inshore and had exchanged shots with them, but they had made their way back into Tripoli despite his efforts, thanks to favorable weather conditions and the protection afforded them by the shoals. Murray wrote in despair that it was hopeless to try to maintain the blockade without plenty of small craft that were able to go into the shallows after the enemy.

On and on ran his complaints. He was running short of food and water. He did not like the thought of trying to maintain the blockade through the winter. He was quite sure the best thing to do was to give up the blockade and buy peace with Tripoli on whatever terms could be obtained.

So one of Morris's captains was writing to him in this vein. Another never wrote at all—Captain George Little

McNeill of the *Boston,* who went wandering off around the Mediterranean without reporting to him. And the other captains all reported that they needed provisions and water—always that need—and often that their ships were in need of repair.

The orders that reached Morris from the Secretary of the Navy were actually three months old and did not lighten his burden at all. The next orders, two and a half months old, increased his burden by ordering home the *Chesapeake* and the *Constellation.*

Meanwhile, Morris's high-spirited officers were quarreling with one another. Stephen Decatur's brother-in-law, a captain of Marines, was killed in a duel with one of the lieutenants of the *Constellation.* That was only one duel out of many. The next development was a duel between Midshipman Joseph Bainbridge and the secretary of the Governor of Malta. The secretary was killed, thanks to Decatur, who as second, insisted that the men should fight at four yards, so close that the inexperienced midshipman could not miss. This was a troublesome triumph, for Morris depended upon Malta for provisions and water and dockyard facilities, and it was hardly tactful to kill the governor's secretary while in need of the hospitality of Malta. It was one more worry for Morris, who had to send Decatur and Bainbridge back to the United States.

Trouble and more trouble! Swedish ships of war and Danish ships of war came sailing up the Mediterranean. They had been sent, apparently, by their governments to bring the Barbary pirates to order, but Morris could not persuade their admirals to make a clear statement regarding their intentions. Having come, they next disappeared without notice, unable to maintain themselves so far from their bases.

The fragile Peace of Amiens, signed by France, England, Spain and Holland, broke up, and half of Europe was at war again. Convoys and privateers and fighting fleets of all nations once more ranged the Mediterranean, and no one knew from one day to another who was neutral and who was at war. The warring nations now had little to spare to help the Americans, and the neutrals were terrified of offending Napoleon and consequently were careful to do nothing at all.

Morris was overwhelmed with troubles. The *Enterprise* needed caulking and re-coppering; the *Chesapeake,* whose mainmast had been defective, now found that her bowsprit was rotten. In spite of everything, Morris continued to convoy American ships. He battled with gales. He sent home the numerous men whose terms of enlistment had expired, and he tried to replace them with others from Mediterranean ports—not easy in a world at war. He transferred himself to the frigate *New York* and within a month the ship was half wrecked as the result of the accidental explosion of some gunpowder below decks. Luckily it was not the main powder store, or Morris and the *New York* would never have been heard of again. As it was, he had to ask help of the Malta dockyard again.

In all the eighteen months Morris was in the Mediterranean he spent scarcely one-tenth of that time fighting the real enemy, Tripoli. There were excuses in plenty for the delays and the inactivity. In war there are always excuses to be found for doing nothing, but wars are won by the men who can think of reasons for action.

The delay at Malta was brightened by the arrival of Captain John Rodgers's small frigate *John Adams* with a prize. It was that same *Meshuda,* once the *Betsey* of Boston, which had lain so long at Gibraltar, and had been weakly allowed to be taken over by the Emperor of Morocco. This ruler showed his gratitude by filling the *Meshuda* with naval stores for Tripoli, but he chose his moment badly. Rodgers, who arrived on the scene unexpectedly, seized her as a blockade runner; she made no attempt to fight.

Perhaps it was this small success that stimulated Morris into activity. The repairs to the *New York* were completed in three weeks, and Morris sailed again for Tripoli with his two frigates and the *Enterprise.* Fortune favored him, and he arrived to find a dozen coasters laden with grain approaching the port. They were convoyed by the Tripolitan gunboats. Morris moved in to the attack, and then hesitated. The gunboats escaped into Tripoli.

The coasters were hauled on shore while a brigade of the Tripolitan army was hurriedly marched out to guard them.

David Porter, lieutenant on the *New York,* pressed for instant action. He wanted to land with a party at once and burn the vessels before the Tripolitans could make them secure. Morris on the quarterdeck of the *New York* eyed the shoals through his telescope—on that treacherous coast his frigates had to lie some miles from the shore— and could not make up his mind. Evening was at hand and he thought it might be better to wait until next day.

During the night the Tripolitan army arrived, and worked like beavers building fortifications out of the sacks of grain from the cargoes. Too late, Morris next morning sent in his boats with Porter in command. A dozen lives were uselessly thrown away. Porter fell wounded. The members of the landing party could not maintain themselves on the beach under the musketry fire from the defenses, and the enemy ships lay too far out for the Americans' gunfire to be effective. Morris transferred his attention from the coasters to the gunboats in Tripoli harbor. He made a feeble thrust at them, and failed again.

It was then, after two failures, that Morris decided to try for peace. He landed under a flag of truce, and the delighted Tripolitans witnessed the spectacle of an American captain, twice repulsed, now offering money to buy a treaty. They could only believe that Morris was moved by fear—there could be no other explanation possible in their minds. Even for us it is hard to understand how Morris could have made such a move; he must have been one of the weakest negotiators that ever was entrusted with American interests.

Congress had authorized Morris to pay up to twenty thousand dollars to secure peace in the Mediterranean. Because he had yet to make treaties with the other Barbary States, he could only offer five thousand dollars to Tripoli. What Tripoli thought of this offer soon became evident. She demanded no less than two hundred thousand dollars in cash and, in addition, repayment of every penny the war had cost her. This demand, if agreed to, gave promise of assuring Tripoli a steady income for years to come.

Morris was utterly crushed by the new failure. He sailed off to Malta again, leaving Rodgers in charge of the blockade. And it was not long before Rodgers had an opportunity to show what stuff he was made of. He kept close in to the port, close enough to notice any unusual movements there. His vigilance was rewarded. Quick eyes at the masthead of the *John Adams* saw the gunboats making preparations for going to sea. Rodgers alerted his three ships and spread them out to bar any possible move. The next morning at dawn he discovered a strange vessel running for Tripoli—she had mistimed her attempt to get in under cover of night.

There was instant action. The *Enterprise* cut the ship off from Tripoli, and she took refuge in a small bay fifteen miles away. Rodgers raced down to the attack. At the same moment the Tripolitan gunboats tried to work their way through the shoals to help their compatriot, and the Tripolitan army marched out hotfoot to play their part.

Rodgers did not waste a moment. Less than three hours after the Tripolitan ship was sighted, the *John Adams* opened fire on her. In that time Rodgers had sailed fifteen miles, worked his ship into the dangerous shoals, and was ready to anchor with "springs" on his cables. This was an arrangement by which he could turn his ship this way and that so as to direct his fire where he wished.

Now the heavy broadside guns of the *John Adams* began to pound the Tripolitan ship, and the latter returned the fire. Cannon smoke drifted around the bay as Rodgers, forbearing to anchor, worked in closer and closer. The well-directed fire was more than the Tripolitans could stand. They hoisted out their boats and fled ashore. At the same moment, the *John Adams,* in danger from rocks and shoals, had to head out again before she could send in her boats to capture the prize.

The Tripolitans started to come back on board their own ship. The Tripolitan army was fast approaching. Rodgers, seeing there was no time to lose, swung the *John Adams* around again and re-opened fire. The cannon shot tore through the ship, and a moment later the Americans were treated to a remarkable display as the Tripolitan ship blew up. Her masts flew a hundred and fifty feet straight up into the air out of the cloud of smoke that engulfed her. When the smoke cleared away there were only fragments floating among the rocks. This was less than four hours after the Tripolitan ship had been sighted. The gunboats hurried back to port, and the army turned around and marched home again.

It had been a brilliant action, well calculated to convince the Tripolitans of the American seamanship and fighting capacity. Now was the moment to press the attack upon the town and compel peace. And this was the moment when Morris's anxieties overcame him. There were no new ones; just the same old troubles of provisions and water, of enlistments expiring and Morocco threatening trouble. He had not even the weather to blame, for this was not yet the end of June, and he could look forward to more than two months of good weather. And yet he abandoned the blockade and sailed away with his squadron on a circular tour of the Western Mediterranean.

The only explanation that can be offered is that Morris found himself unable to support any longer the burden of his responsibilities. He may have been in such a mood that he could persuade himself that he had accomplished his task, or he may have thought that the task was one that could never be accomplished.

Off he went, through the lovely Straits of Messina, into the beautiful Bay of Naples. He conferred with the Minister of the King of Naples regarding the loan of small craft, and the possibility of using Neapolitan dockyards. The Neapolitan government was probably the most corrupt and inefficient in Europe, but its help might be better than nothing. That help was not offered very readily, because Naples was hesitating on the brink of entering into the war on one side or the other.

From Naples Morris proceeded slowly toward Gibraltar. When he was nearly there he received an order from the Secretary of the Navy removing him from his command. Morris was one of the few men who was at all surprised at such an action. His unhappy story ends with a court of inquiry and his dismissal from the Navy. It was a severe sentence, in fact a brutal one, especially as he had no opportunity of excusing himself before a court-martial. He paid, in fact, for the disappointment of the high hopes with which America had sent him out eighteen months before. Perhaps the severity of his treatment was a hint of the determination of the administration to fight the war with new energy.

# CHAPTER 5

# *PHILADELPHIA AGROUND—*
# *307 PRISONERS TAKEN*

MR. JEFFERSON AND THE SECRETARY OF THE
Navy, Mr. Robert Smith, were indeed set on fighting to a
finish. Man of peace though Jefferson was, and even
though the cost of the war was appalling to his frugal
mind, he was determined to go ahead. Morris's complaints about the lack of small craft resulted in Congress's voting the sum of ninety-six thousand dollars to
build two schooners and two brigs. These were the
famous ships the *Nautilus* and the *Vixen,* the *Argus* and
the *Syren.*

The United States government was now acting vigorously. It might be thought that the Louisiana Purchase, which had just been completed, had given the nation new life. Now that her destiny of expansion was settled, the United States was determined to take her rightful place among the nations of the world.

Ships were being refitted, new crews were being recruited, and, most important of all, a new commander had been selected. Edward Preble was one of the most junior captains, a fact which caused constant trouble.

Seniority meant much in the United States Navy, as in all fighting services. In war one man can give orders to another which will send that man into deadly peril, perhaps to his death. And those orders are given by virtue of the fact that one man's commission bears a date perhaps only a few days earlier than the other's. Those orders are given, too, in the certainty of instant obedience; disobedience (although the fact is rarely mentioned) may be paid for by a shameful death before an execution squad. So seniority is of vast importance. Moreover, every officer of a fighting service who is worth

65

his salt is burning to distinguish himself. He will resent bitterly the appointment of a man junior to himself to a position that he might have had himself.

So seniority is not a matter to be treated lightly. No country has ever found it easy to put a senior under a junior's orders. Yet every country has to face the problem that an officer may be promoted and acquire seniority before there has been a chance to find out whether he is fit for high command.

The large navies of other countries solved this problem by promoting every captain in his turn to admiral and then leaving the unsatisfactory admirals unemployed or giving them administrative posts where they could do no harm. But America had no admirals (the title sounded undemocratic) and few enough captains, and administrative posts of any dignity did not exist.

The appointment of Preble to the command in the Mediterranean meant the recall of every captain senior to him, including the active and brilliant Rodgers. It also meant, that when the Mediterranean squadron was reinforced to the point where more captains were needed than there were captains junior to Preble, Preble had to give up the command. It was the price that had to be paid for discipline and order, and even Jefferson's genius could not devise a way around the difficulty.

After the removal of Morris, however, Preble was in command. He sailed in August, 1803, in the *Constitution,* arrived at Gibraltar in September, and made his personality and ability instantly felt throughout the squadron. So far, he was almost unknown to his brother officers, except by reputation as the man who in command of the *Essex* had sailed to Batavia and back without losing a single man from sickness. He had convoyed on that occasion an American merchant fleet halfway round the world to the romantic Spice Islands. His success had made him known among merchant skippers, but not among his brother captains, for he had been out of all contact with them for a year. But they soon learned to know him better, with his stern but just discipline, his abounding energy, his capacity for organization, and his fearless acceptance of responsibility. The peppery-tempered unknown soon became the beloved commander, and the American squadron at once became a force to be feared. Preble was like a skilled teamster taking over the reins after a clumsy driver had unsettled the horses; he had his team at once in hand and pulling vigorously and together.

And credit must be given to Jefferson and Robert Smith. It was they who had named Preble to the command; it was they who issued his orders, and it was they who chiefly selected the brilliant band of young officers who served under him. The victories of 1812 were mostly won by men who had been trained by Preble. Yet many of those men were first selected and put in the way of distinction by Mr. Robert Smith during Mr. Jefferson's administration.

The arrival of Preble and his ships brought an instant change in the North African situation. He struck at once at the nearest enemy. The Emperor of Morocco arrived at Tangier to find a powerful American squadron anchored in the port, their decks cleared for action and guns run out. The Moroccan ships of war were in American hands, their officers and crews were American prisoners, and it only needed a word from Preble to lay Tangier in ruins.

Preble had seized the right moment and the perfect opportunity to bring pressure on Morocco. Tangier was the most vulnerable of all the North African ports and Preble had the largest possible force in hand.

The Emperor had to yield at once, and there was a rapid change from war to peace, from hatred to friendship. The United States had never had such a good friend as the Empire of Morocco, declared the Emperor. The Moorish warships which had gone out to take prizes (and had fallen into American hands) had not been obeying his orders, but those of the Governor of Tangier, who would be punished for his behavior. The American ships must need fresh provisions. Here were live cattle and sheep and fowls, as a gift, not for sale. Surely now it would be easy to come to terms?

Easy enough, Preble replied, as long as those terms were his own. He demanded an instant declaration of peace with not a penny paid for it. There would not even be a present for the prime minister. Preble also demanded a mutual exchange of prisoners and prizes.

The Emperor agreed; the American prisoners were released, and the Moroccan vessels handed back. Peace was solemnly declared and salutes given and returned to ratify it. Now Preble could sail away with his free livestock on board.

There was still work to be done at the Gibraltar end of the Mediterranean. There were American ships to be convoyed. The blockade of Tripoli had to be reproclaimed to undo the work of Morris, one of whose last acts had been (yielding to Moroccan threats) to permit grain vessels free entry to Tripoli. Arrangements had to be made for American storeships to come far up the Mediterranean instead of stopping at Gibraltar as their previous contracts had agreed. But none of this was to delay for a moment the new blockade of Tripoli. Captain William Bainbridge had already been sent with the *Philadelphia* and *Vixen* to take station outside that port.

Preble dealt with his numerous affairs, established his line of communication, and started after him.

Then, early one morning, with the mountains of Sardinia in sight, the topsails of a frigate came up over the horizon. She was British—H.M.S. *Amazon*—and she sent up a signal to say that she had important news. It was appalling news.

The *Amazon* had just come from Malta. Before she left, the Danish consul there had received a letter from the Danish consul at Tripoli, telling that the *Philadelphia* had been captured. Bainbridge and three hundred and seven officers and men, and a fine frigate, were in the hands of the Tripolitan pirates. It was "melancholy and distressing intelligence," as Preble said in his report. He pushed on to Malta to hear the details, and Bainbridge's report awaited him there.

It was one of those disasters made possible only by a whole series of coincidences. Bainbridge, from his station off Tripoli, had sent the *Vixen* westward to intercept two corsairs that he had heard were cruising in that direction. Alone, he maintained the blockade until a westerly gale blew him away from the port. When the wind shifted and he was returning, he sighted a Tripolitan ship which was sneaking into the harbor. Bainbridge hurried to the attack, pressing in among the dangerous and unknown shallows, his guns firing at long range. From little platforms at the sides of the ship, he had men heaving the lead, constantly lowering over the side weights attached to lines by which they could tell the depths of water under the ship.

The Tripolitan ship had too good a start. She slipped into the harbor just in time and Bainbridge turned away, having penetrated to the very mouth of the harbor. The minarets and towers of Tripoli were plainly in view under the noontime sun. At that moment Lieutenant David Porter (newly recovered from his wounds) was by Bainbridge's orders climbing the rigging of the mizzen mast so as to be able to see what other ships the Tripolitans had in harbor, and in what state of readiness.

The lead was hauled up ready to be cast again. Before it could drop—before Porter could reach the masthead—

there was a shattering crash and a mighty jerk as the *Philadelphia* reared up and stopped, her bows inclined upwards, and leaning heavily over to one side. The *Philadelphia* was fast aground on the Kaliusa reef, well known of course to the Tripolitans but not marked on any chart that Bainbridge had. He had taken every possible precaution he could without being timid, and this disaster had befallen him.

He did all he could to get his ship free. He turned his sails against the wind in an attempt to back the ship off the rocks. He set his men to work in furious haste on the heeling deck to lighten her so that she might float. Everything was flung over the side: the anchors and then the guns, save for one or two that might be used to defend the ship against attack. The pumps were set to work, pumping the precious drinking water into the sea.

It was of no use; the bow had run too far up onto the rocks—she lay there in only twelve feet of water. There was one last sacrifice that could be made. Axes were brought and the shrouds that supported the foremast were cut. As soon as they parted the mast fell over the

73

side, so greatly was the ship heeled over. The foremast was of great weight, and of course losing it relieved the ship in the part that was most aground, but the loss did not set her free. She was still hard and fast on the rocks, and nothing, it seemed, would float her off.

Nor was all this work performed without interference. The delighted Tripolitans, as soon as they saw what had happened, manned their gunboats and swarmed out to the attack. They were only little boats, but that meant they could be easily moved with oars. The one or two guns they carried were very heavy and powerful, capable of sending a shot through the side of any ship in the world. The Tripolitans came rowing out across the harbor, clustered under the stern of the helpless ship, and opened a slow but methodical fire.

Bainbridge could do nothing in reply. His ship had fallen so far over on one side, and the bows were forced so high, that he could not use the guns he had left, especially as the Tripolitans chose to attack on the quarter. This was the angle between the stern and the side, where ships of that day, even when on an even keel, found difficulty in bringing guns into action. Bainbridge hauled a gun or two to the threatened point, and had his men bring their axes there and actually cut away part of the side of the ship to try to return the fire. He found, however, that this was impossible on a deck that pointed to the sky.

It was part of Bainbridge's bad luck that he had sent the *Vixen* away. Had she been with him she would probably have been used in the chase, and the *Philadelphia* would not have gone aground at all. Even with the *Philadelphia* aground, the *Vixen* would have kept the gunboats at a distance and prevented any attack from the shore, so that Bainbridge could have floated his ship off. As it was, he had no chance.

The gunboats continued their monotonous pounding. For six hours the men had toiled without success to free the ship, and darkness was approaching. But not darkness only. The Tripolitan army of several thousand men was ready by now. There were scores of small boats available to carry them out to the wreck, and the few guns left would not be able to fire on them. In the darkness an attack would be launched with odds of ten to one, and there would be massacre and murder.

Bainbridge fulfilled his last duty. The pumps were set to work again, pumping water onto the gunpowder in the magazines. Everything that might be of value to a warlike power—the muskets, the cutlasses—was thrown overboard, and the carpenter was sent down to bore holes in the bottom of the ship. And then, just after the flaming sun had set, and as the attack gathered strength, Bainbridge hauled down the flag.

The Tripolitans swarmed on board, mad as usual for personal plunder. They stripped the wretched prisoners of their clothes before bringing them ashore. There was a surf breaking on the beach and the Americans were forced to wade in through it, to where the Tripolitan army was waiting for them. Then the Americans were marched to their prison—a dirty warehouse which they had to clean out before it was fit for habitation, and so small that there was not floor space for them all to lie down at once. Not until the evening of the next day did anyone think of giving them anything to eat.

Bainbridge and his officers were led in triumph through the marble halls of the palace, before the Pasha on his throne, and then confined in the house which until a short time before had been occupied by the American consul.

But there was much more to add to their unhappiness. Two days after the surrender a brisk wind came blowing in from the sea. It piled the water up on the reef to increase the depth, and helped the thousands of men who were set to work to recover the ship. Anchors were laid out astern of her with cables leading to the ship, and the Tripolitans labored at the capstan to haul her off. The gunboats pulled with all the strength of their rowers, and eventually the *Philadelphia* came free.

In a sheltered harbor, with plenty of skilled labor at hand, the leaks in the vessel's bottom could be easily dealt with. Tripoli now had in her possession the finest frigate she had ever owned, built by Josiah Fox to the order of the city after which she was named, as a gift to the United States.

Nor was that all. The guns and weapons which Bainbridge had thrown overboard lay on the rocks in less than twenty feet of water. There were plenty of coral divers and sponge fishers in Tripoli to whom twenty feet of water was a trifle. It was not long before the guns were mounted again on the *Philadelphia* and the ship was once more a dangerous fighting vessel. The prisoners, when they were marched to work on the fortifications, could look out unhappily across the harbor and see the *Philadelphia* riding to her anchor with the Tripolitan flag at her peak.

It was a state of affairs that enormously complicated Preble's task. He was under orders not only to make war on Tripoli but also to negotiate a peace. And now Tripoli had in her possession bargaining counters of great value. No doubt the pirates would put up their price. They had won a decided victory, and, even though luck had given it to them, it was only natural that they might think they could win others. It was possible that they might, by actual ill-treatment of the prisoners, put pressure on Preble to hasten the conclusion of peace. Even if they did not do so deliberately it was not pleasant for Preble to think about the three hundred Americans in enemy hands.

It was usual, in those days, for a nation to give the prisoners that it took the same rations and treatment that it gave its own fighting men. (Later on the practice became the subject of treaties between various countries.) But the Tripolitan seaman was never properly fed or clothed by his government, so that Bainbridge's men could expect to be starved and cold and verminous, as indeed they were. Preble knew that should he refuse the terms demanded by Tripoli he was prolonging and perhaps increasing the misery suffered by his fellow countrymen.

The capture of the *Philadelphia* introduced another complication, for it gave the pirates a vessel of speed and power. There was always the chance that they might man her and bring her out to fight, and in all Preble's squadron there was only the *Constitution* that could hope to meet her with any chance of success. It was a possibility that always had to be borne in mind; one more anxiety for Preble.

He dealt with his problems without any delay. He found food and water for his ships. Through the British consul he was able to send money and clothing to Bainbridge for the use of the prisoners. He re-rigged the *Syren,* for the shipbuilders in the yard had tried to improve on her design and had injured her sailing qualities thereby. He made an inquiry of the Tripolitan agent at Malta regarding peace terms, and sheered off abruptly when he heard that the first item was a demand by Tripoli for a complete schooner of war in exchange for the *Philadelphia.*

Preble went down to Tripoli with his squadron and for the first time in his life he examined the place with his own eyes. It was probably then that he began to form the plan that he carried out so brilliantly shortly afterwards. And of course he tightened up the blockade of the port, weathering the winter gales and capturing, to the vast annoyance of the Pasha, the ketch *Mastico,* a small two-masted sailing ship. It was carrying presents—among them forty-two African slaves—for the Ottoman government at Constantinople.

Here was one of the small craft so urgently needed for inshore fighting. Preble took the *Mastico* into the American service. He had to give her a new name. No one knows now just why he selected the name *Intrepid,* but whether the choice was casual or not it added a glorious name to the records of American naval history.

# CHAPTER 6

# DECATUR DESTROYS THE
## *PHILADELPHIA*

PREBLE WAS ALREADY RESOLVED THAT THE
*Philadelphia* must be destroyed. Probably he had decided
on that as soon as he heard the news of her loss, before
even he gazed at her through his telescope as the *Constitution* beat about outside the harbor. He had only to
decide upon a plan of action, one that had a chance of
success, at whatever cost.

Bainbridge, in prison, had written to him in invisible
ink suggesting such an attempt. Now Stephen Decatur,
who had been sent back to the Mediterranean and was
captain of the *Enterprise,* came to him with suggestions.

And immediately afterwards, Lieutenant Charles Stewart, commanding the *Syren,* also asked for an interview and proposed an attack on the *Philadelphia.* It was only natural that every officer and man in the squadron should wish to redeem her loss.

The ideal, of course, would be to recapture her, bring her out from Tripoli and hoist the Stars and Stripes once more on board her. In naval history there were plenty of examples of similar feats, and during the then current war between France and England new ones were being continually added. The usual plan was to send in a large attacking force by night in boats, to board the vessel, overpower her crew, and come sailing out with the prize. Preble must have thought longingly of doing the same, and yet he rejected the scheme. There might be three hundred, there might be five hundred, men on board the *Philadelphia,* and the total number of men under his own command was less than a thousand. It would be hard to send in a force that could be certain of seizing the *Philadelphia* and at the same time retain enough men to man his own ships adequately.

Besides, a force of three hundred men would fill seven or eight boats, and seven or eight boats could not hope to escape detection while rowing all the way up into Tripoli harbor. An alarm, an early warning to the *Philadelphia,* would deprive the boarding party of the advantage of

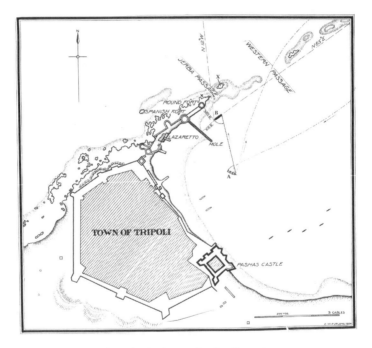

**Historical Chart of Tripoli Harbor**
*"A" marks* Philadelphia*'s position when boarded by Decatur's men from the* Intrepid, *16 February, 1804.*
*"B" is the location of her wreck.*
*"X" (just west of the Jerba Passage) is the location of the* Intrepid*'s wreck after she blew up on 4 September 1804, during another mission into Tripoli harbor.*

surprise and would result in a long fight. That could bring about both the arrival of reinforcements from the Tripolitan army on shore and also the battering by the guns of the defenses of the ship if captured.

Preble saw clearly that the attempt must not fail. Another defeat, another repulse, would mean that negotiations with Tripoli for any reasonable terms of peace would be impossible. It might also have a depressing effect on his own forces, although now that Preble was coming to know the young men under his command he thought he could put that fear aside.

But it was a long, long way out to the gap in the reef from where the *Philadelphia* lay at anchor. A wind that would carry an attacking force in would work against them when they tried to sail the *Philadelphia* out. Furthermore, the Tripolitans had not yet replaced the foremast Bainbridge had cut away. Perhaps, thought Preble, his men could tow the *Philadelphia* out with boats. No, that would take a long time—a full hour. All that time the batteries could fire on the fragile boats towing, and the Tripolitan gunboats could cut them off.

No, there was too little hope of bringing the *Philadel-phia* out, and this was not the moment to take a very big risk. Preble, sitting in his cabin or walking his quarterdeck—already tortured by the disease that was to kill him a few years later—had to discard the idea.

So if the *Philadelphia* could not be brought out she must be destroyed. That would be risky enough, but it was a risk worth taking. That meant setting her on fire—wooden ships were hard to sink but easy to burn. The timbers were weathered and covered with paint; the rigging was tarred—flame would run up a burning rope like a firework. The sails were great masses of dry canvas, and then there was the powder magazine; it would take only a single spark there to blow the ship to fragments. Fire was the most constant danger in the old ships, and strict rules were enforced about lights on board. If a determined body of men set the *Philadelphia* thoroughly on fire she was doomed.

But it could only be a small body of men; that was already plain, for it was absolutely necessary to achieve surprise. Those men must get on board without causing an alarm to be given. It could be done by use of clever disguise. The thought of disguise called to Preble's mind the captured *Mastico*—the new *Intrepid*. There she was, looking like all the hundreds of other small coasters to be found in the inlets of North Africa. She might come in unquestioned, sneaking in at night like any other blockade runner. Then she could drift alongside the *Philadelphia,* and determined men could do the rest. There would be other advantages in using the *Intrepid*. She was small enough to be moved by oars—the long sweeps that every North African craft employed—so that she could get out again without depending on the wind. That would give her crew at least a chance of escape. Preble of course did not want his men to lose their lives, nor did he want to see another batch of captives added to the three hundred that Tripoli already held prisoner. But being small, the *Intrepid* could carry only a small force. Preble called in Decatur and discussed the question again.

Decatur undertook the mission, naturally, eagerly. Stewart was disappointed. It was his hard luck that Decatur had had first opportunity of discussing the mission with Preble. That gave Decatur the right to try it, together with the opportunity of distinguishing himself, and the chance of being killed. Every man in Decatur's *Enterprise* volunteered. Decatur took sixty-two of them. Also included in the party were his own officers, five midshipmen from the *Constitution,* and—may his name be remembered—a Sicilian named Salvatore Catalano, who served with the squadron as pilot.

The *Intrepid* was sixty feet long (there are plenty of pleasure yachts larger than that), and the seventy-four men crammed themselves on board. The *Constitution,* the *Intrepid,* the *Enterprise,* and the *Syren* were lying in Syracuse harbor in Sicily at the time, and there every man was drilled in the part he was to play. Every man knew what he had to do once the *Intrepid* was alongside the *Philadelphia.* Preble's written orders to Decatur went into great detail regarding exactly how the ship was to be set on fire. This was a sign of the anxiety Preble felt, as otherwise he would have left a free hand to that very capable officer, Decatur.

So off went the *Intrepid* with the *Syren* under Stewart's command to accompany her. The men on board were crammed so close that midshipmen and marines shared the privilege of sleeping on top of the water casks in the hold. They were packed like sardines— and at the same time devoured by the vermin left in the ship by the former African owners. They ate the stores found in the ship, too, and the food was stinking and rotten. But it was only four days' easy sail from Syracuse to Tripoli, and they could endure four days of discomfort.

The night of their arrival a roaring westerly wind such as one might expect in February blew them far to the eastward. This forced the men to endure nine days more as they beat back to the harbor—nine days more of cramp and suffocation, vermin and food poisoning. At last they crawled back to Tripoli, and sighted the place with a gentle northerly wind blowing. The *Intrepid* took the lead, and the *Syren* held back so as not to appear to be acquainted.

The Americans looking out from their prison saw the two vessels and wondered what they were. The *Syren* was far distant, and no one recognized her; what with the convoy work she had undertaken and the alterations carried out in Malta, she was unknown at Tripoli. The *Intrepid* was obviously a merchant ship, and William Ray, the captured marine whose diary tells us much about what went on in Tripoli, thought that she might be bringing in envoys to discuss peace. What he did not know, and what Preble's intelligence service had discovered, was that the Tripolitans had recently bought at Malta a two-masted vessel rigged like the *Syren,* and were expecting her arrival.

The wind was dropping now and night was approaching. It had been agreed in the original plan that the *Intrepid* was to be reinforced by the boats and boats' crews of the *Syren,* but Decatur decided that he would not wait for them. By a fortunate chance he had taken over one of the *Syren's* boats the day before, and it was towing astern. His timing was excellent. Without appearing to delay, he had reached the entrance to the harbor just after nightfall, and by the light of the moon he was able to steer for the *Philadelphia.*

He and Catalano and one or two more were visible on deck wearing Turkish clothing; the others were lying out of sight, flat on the deck or huddled in the hold. The wind carried the boat ever so slowly toward the *Philadelphia,* with Catalano steering.

The Tripolitan crew were taking the evening air on deck, idly watching the *Intrepid* approaching. They hailed to warn her to keep clear, but Catalano hailed back in *lingua franca,* the mixture of all the languages spoken round the Mediterranean. A Turk would use it when speaking to a Berber.

Catalano was ready with his story—it had long been thought out. He said his ship had lost her anchors, and asked permission to tie up alongside the *Philadelphia* for the night. Permission was granted without a thought, and a word or two of gossip exchanged. Catalano's statement that the brig outside was the *Transfer*—that was the name of the brig which the Tripolitans had just bought at Malta—gave the final touch of reality.

When the two vessels were only twenty yards apart, the wind failed. This left the *Intrepid* lying helpless, with the seventy men of her crew hardly daring to breathe as they lay tightly packed on the planking. As in any other military plan, however well devised, something unexpected had happened, and bold action, clear-headed action, was necessary. At a murmured order from Decatur, the men in Turkish dress climbed down into the *Syren's* boat, which was mercifully towing astern. Slowly and leisurely it had to be done, however desperate the moment, because haste and smartness would be suspicious.

By the time the Americans had taken a rope from the *Intrepid's* bow, the *Philadelphia* had obligingly sent off her boat with a rope too. After the two ropes were fastened together, the boats returned to their respective ships. The men in sight on the deck began to haul in on the rope; those lying down seized it and gave what help they could. Then the *Intrepid* began to close the gap between the ships, inch by inch and yard by yard. The sides of the vessels were about to touch when a cry of alarm went up from the *Philadelphia.*

"Board!" said Decatur, and the Americans sprang to their feet, weapons in hand, and clambered up the side of the *Philadelphia.* It was a complete surprise; not one Tripolitan had time to seize musket or pistol as the wave of Americans swept along the decks. Not a shot was fired. One American received a wound; a score of Tripolitans who tried to show fight or who were too stupefied to run were cut down.

Decatur led the final charge on the Tripolitans huddled together in the bows. He swept them overboard—into the sea or down into their boat.

Already the rest of the plan was under way. The Americans who had been detailed to remain in the *Intrepid* were passing out oily rags, bundles of straw and oakum soaked in turpentine—everything for a quick, fierce blaze. The boarding parties took them and hurried them to the cockpit and the storerooms and the berth deck.

The glowing slow matches were whirled round until they were burning brightly, and then were thrust into the heaps.

In the cramped quarters of a wooden ship a heap of straw blazing on one deck would have the deck above on fire in a moment; with the hatchways and ports all open there was plenty of draft. It was scarcely a matter of seconds before the whole ship was full of roaring flames. So quickly did they spread that one or two Americans were nearly cut off by them. But everyone succeeded in tumbling back on board—they even dragged back with them one unhappy Tripolitan prisoner. Then they cut the ropes and shoved the *Intrepid* clear.

There was desperate need for haste because on the *Intrepid*'s deck were plenty more combustibles, piled there in case Decatur should see an opportunity of using the *Intrepid* as a fireship. A spark from the blazing inferno which the *Philadelphia* had become would send the *Intrepid* up in flames as well. This was not a time for further risks, so the crew, remembering their drill, began

94

to row the *Intrepid* away. Although they worked hard, with long, long pulls at the clumsy oars, their movements seemed painfully slow, but the *Intrepid* gradually gathered way.

It took time to cover any distance. Luckily, it also took time for the Tripolitans to come to their senses, for the sleeping garrison on shore to wake up and get to their guns, for the crews of the other ships to hoist up their anchors. Most of the firing came from the *Philadelphia's* own guns, which were loaded and went off one by one as the flames reached them. The flames were already roaring up the rigging. They reached the cables that secured the vessel and burned them through, so that the frigate for a little while drifted in the harbor.

At last the fire reached the magazine and the explosion blew the ship to fragments, which rained down into the harbor. Some of the fragments were dredged up from the bottom forty years later by an American captain.

Stewart, in the *Syren* outside the harbor, saw the blaze and knew that the attack had gained its objective. He saw the explosion, and then, long minutes afterwards, he saw the rocket which Decatur sent up. It announced that the *Intrepid* had escaped and gave notice of her location. Stewart sent in his boats to help her, and soon Decatur stepped on board the *Syren* to report to his superior.

It was not for long that Stewart would be Decatur's superior, for Decatur was promoted to captain over Stewart's head as soon as the news of the *Philadelphia's* destruction reached America. That was the fortune of war, and Stewart had to be content with promotion to the rank of Master Commandant, newly revived by Congress.

As if to make up for the tricks it had played previously, the wind now freshened and blew from the right quarter. It was only for three nights and two days that the seventy men in the *Intrepid* had to endure overcrowding and fleas and poisonous food.

Preble, waiting at Syracuse in the *Constitution,* with the *Vixen* and the *Enterprise* anchored beside him, saw the two ships coming up over the horizon, sixteen days after they had set out. We can only guess how long those sixteen days had seemed to Preble. The grim, lean old man, with what was left of his once red hair already gray, heard the news that his plan had been completely successful. Not a life had been lost, and there was nothing left of the *Philadelphia*.

# CHAPTER 7

# U.S. MAINTAINS FRAGILE BLOCKADE

THE BURNING OF THE *PHILADELPHIA* WAS A load off Preble's mind; but Preble's mind bore many loads. Although he was free now from the nightmare possibility of the Tripolitans sailing out in the *Philadelphia,* he still had plenty to think about. There was the blockade to be maintained, through the wild winter weather, and he maintained it, although storms damaged his ships and presented him with the fresh problem of how to get them repaired. That the blockade was effective was proved by the prizes that he took.

Yet those prizes meant more reports to be written and

more responsibility, for a blockade always brings about trouble with the neutrals whose business is being interfered with and whose property is being seized. Many times in her history America has been the neutral, and has naturally experienced a sense of grievance at her losses. At that very moment United States shipping was suffering because of the war between England and Napoleon. The same thing would happen again in 1916 when England would be at war with Germany.

Of course, the United States has felt differently when she has been the blockading power. During the Civil War the American Navy enforced the blockade of Southern ports as rigorously as any blockade has ever been enforced. And in 1917 when the United States declared war on Germany she tightened up the rules against which she had protested the year before.

The United States was the blockading power in 1806 in the Mediterranean, and Preble enforced her rights, seizing ships of any nationality that tried to run either inward or outward through the blockade he had proclaimed. He was fully entitled to do so, especially as he took care to maintain the blockade day after day. (By international law a blockade must be constant and maintained in force.) But the sufferers protested. Morocco and Tunis and Algiers neither liked the thought of their fellow Muslims being under blockade nor wished to lose the profits resulting from the transport of foodstuffs to Tripoli.

The owners of other captured ships protested to their governments and threatened to bring suit against Preble in the Federal Courts for damages. There was a Russian ship which Stewart caught trying to escape from Tripoli. Preble could have made a prize of her, but he let her go. He knew that the Czar of Russia was a man of uncertain temper who believed he had great interests in the Mediterranean. He laid claim to rule over Malta, and had a powerful fleet in the Mediterranean at that moment. Preble, rather than risk offending a freakish monarch who had seven battleships close at hand, gave up the prize. It must be remembered that under the old laws, Preble received a share of the value of every prize taken.

Giving up the Russian ship was a sensible act, but it meant more letters, reports and decisions.

Another source of trouble was the King of Naples, who had to be persuaded to lend gunboats and crews for the attack on Tripoli that Preble intended. The King, with his kingdom trembling on the brink of disaster (less than two years later Napoleon seized half his dominions), was a man who found it hard to make up his mind. Preble had to write many letters and use much persuasion to bring him to a decision.

Then there was the eternal question of food and water. Preble was at liberty to purchase stores from Sicily, but that was the most misgoverned corner of Europe (under the same King of Naples). And although it was hard to find stores there, it was harder still to meet the prices that were asked by the Sicilians during the wartime shortages. Stores sent out from America were at least two months old when they reached him, and we find Preble reporting that a large amount had to be thrown overboard as useless upon arrival.

To add to his troubles, the terms of enlistment of his men were expiring. That had to be attended to and more men found and trained. Of course, like every officer commanding any fleet anywhere in the world, he was plagued by the desertion of some of his seamen.

Life on board a ship of war was desperately hard, and when the opportunity came, many men tried to escape. This was especially true of those men who had incurred the dislike of some officer and who faced a future of repeated floggings. (It was 1861 before flogging was abolished in the United States Navy.) That being the case, it was better to escape even into another ship of war to start afresh. It was certainly better to escape into a merchant ship where the pay was far higher and conditions not so severe.

Seamen in general were literally a floating population, with no home ties, and no families. They spent their hard brief lives in one ship after another, quite unfitted for any life on shore. It hardly mattered to them which country they served or under which flag they sailed. So American seamen deserted to British ships, and British seamen deserted to American ships. This was, of course, trouble-some to the captains who lost their services and had to try to replace them.

Preble made use of Sicilian ports rather than British because of this very problem of desertion. In Sicily there were not so many ships to desert into and with most of his men the difference of language discouraged deser-tion to the shore. It meant trouble one way or the other in any case.

# CHAPTER 8

# PREBLE ATTACKS TRIPOLI!

UNDER THE BLUE SKY LAY THE VIVID COLORS of the Mediterranean. Far out the sea was a blue even more intense than the sky, but nearer in the blue abruptly changed to a clear green, and beyond that the green shaded into yellow, marking the shoals that made this coast so dangerous. A line of jagged rocks, gray and black and red, constituted more obvious dangers to ships venturing in.

On the far side of the rocks stretched the shore line, low and level, in color a yellowish sandy gray, but so low that for a little way out to sea it was invisible. Yet it could still be traced by the palm trees that extended along it, their feathery tops spaced out all along the horizon.

There was nothing remarkable about the coast except for the city that stood there, with the palms extending on either side of it. Gleaming white in the sunshine lay the city within its bastioned walls. Above it towered the castle, a hundred and fifty feet high, solidly built in its lower stories but arched and airy in the upper ones. From the flagstaff above it the flag of Tripoli fluttered in the gentle land breeze.

On that blazing afternoon the little harbor was a scene of furious activity. Cannons were roaring and booming in a continuous rolling of gunfire, and powder smoke was drifting in dense banks over the sea. Men were fighting desperately for their lives and honor amid the shafts of sunlight that pierced the powder smoke.

Commodore Preble was delivering his attack upon Tripoli. There was to be an end of simple blockade, of negotiations, and of threats. Vigorous action might bring the pirates to their senses. Preble had assembled every ship and every man available for this assault, but the sum total of ships and men was neither great nor terrifying. Of ships there were a single frigate, half a dozen little brigs and schooners no bigger than a wealthy man's yacht, and eight clumsy gun vessels that were smaller still. The total of all the crews was only a thousand men, and of these a hundred were Neapolitans borrowed from the King of Naples to help man the borrowed gun vessels.

To oppose this small force, Tripoli had her light craft with nearly as many men as Preble had under his command, and she had manned her shore batteries of a hundred heavy guns with thousands of gunners. Preble was embarking upon a desperate venture in attempting to take wooden ships in against those stone walls, and amid those rocks and shoals. However, if skill and courage could gain a victory in the face of such odds, the skill and courage were available. The list of the junior officers is studded with names destined for immortality. Decatur and Stewart, James Lawrence and Thomas Macdonough were only a few among the many young and vigorous men burning for distinction and reckless of their lives.

Stephen Decatur took his division of three gunboats in among the Tripolitan light vessels where they sheltered among the shoals. Outnumbered in boats and vastly outnumbered in men, he attacked with a dash and ferocity that the Barbary pirates could not match. He took his own gunboat alongside a Tripolitan and boarded her. Sixteen men followed him with ax and pike, pistol and cutlass. There were thirty-six of the enemy, but the wild attack gave them no chance. Sixteen were killed and fifteen wounded before the remaining five had time to surrender.

Decatur was towing the Tripolitan vessel away as a prize when he heard that his brother had just been mortally wounded by a pirate who had pretended to surrender. The news helped to keep his fighting fury at a white heat. A moment later he was alongside another Tripolitan gunboat—whether the assassin's or not, no one can be sure—and a moment after that, he was leaping on her deck with Macdonough and the remnant of his crew following him. There were twenty-four Tripolitans to oppose him, headed by their burly captain. Decatur's cutlass broke off at the hilt when it clashed against the Tripolitan's pike. Undaunted, Decatur grappled and fell with his man, and shot him with a pistol which he did not draw from his pocket but fired through the cloth of his coat. The raging Americans then went storming on into the crowded boat. Three unwounded Tripolitans surrendered; four more were wounded but lived, and the other seventeen were dead.

Decatur brought out his two prizes; Lieutenant John Trippe had brought out another.

Meanwhile Preble had come boldly in with the *Constitution*, tacking and weaving so that his guns could sweep every part of the Tripolitan defenses in turn. The batteries he fired at promptly ceased their fire as the gunners ducked behind cover, and as promptly opened fire again as he turned away. Preble's grapeshot swept away the crews of some of the gunboats. These men were promptly replaced from the waiting hundreds on shore. But his round-shot sank two or three of the gunboats.

Meanwhile his two "mortar vessels" had been trying to throw shells into the city. The "mortar vessels" were Neapolitan ships, with Neapolitan shells, and not very effective. The shells scared most of the civilian population out into the surrounding country, and damaged a good many houses, including that of the Danish consul—an innocent bystander if ever there was one.

So the sultry afternoon wore on—an afternoon in Africa in August, with the cannon thundering over the water and the great banks of powder smoke drifting in the slight breeze. But there was a special significance about the drifting of that smoke. It was beginning to blow into shore. The wind was veering around, blowing from sea to land, as is always likely to happen in hot latitudes in the afternoon. Every moment made it more difficult to keep the wind from sweeping the American sailing ships toward that dangerous shore. If a ship should be disabled the task would be nearly impossible—

and already the *Constitution* had one shot clean through her mainmast.

Preble hoisted the signal that told his small fleet to leave the scene of action. As he swung his ship around he let loose with a couple of final broadsides. They brought down the minaret of the mosque, a Muslim house of prayer and worship that towered beside the castle.

The little squadron worked its way clear, prizes and all, and gathered round the flagship out at sea. But there could be no question of resting. Every officer and man fell to work preparing for a new attack, urged on not only by Preble's orders but by his own desire to give the enemy no time to recover. All the ships were much cut about in their rigging; new sails had to be bent and new ropes rove. The three prizes were re-rigged completely and crews allotted to them. Ammunition and provisions had to be distributed.

The work was finished in less than forty-eight hours. Then in went the squadron again, cannon thundering, officers walking the decks with the enemy's shot howling overhead, gun crews toiling in the heat with tackles and rammers, and powder boys running about with cartridges.

The enemy had learned from experience. This time more of their light craft came to grips with the Americans, and the guns were better aimed. Probably the Pasha of Tripoli (the Bashaw, as Preble spelt his title, with a much better attempt at the pronunciation) had been threatening to take off a few heads if more damage were not done to the enemy. The American gunboats were badly battered and one of them blew up. After three hours of furious fighting Preble drew off again as the wind worked around.

That night he received crushing news. The frigate *John Adams* had arrived while the action was at its height. She was not of much use as a reinforcement, for most of her guns were unmounted to make room for the stores she carried. Far worse, she carried dispatches to say that Preble was being superseded in his command. Commodore Samuel Barron was on his way with four additional frigates; and as there were only two more captains on the Navy List junior to Preble, the command had to be given to an officer senior to him. It was a bitter blow to Preble, who had been in command for a whole year in the Mediterranean, bearing heavy responsibilities and struggling against endless difficulties.

Nor was this all—not by any means. Preble had no way of knowing when Barron would arrive, and meanwhile the summer was coming to an end. This was August, and by September bad weather might be expected, with northerly gales that would make the coast even more dangerous. It was Preble's duty to shoulder the responsibility and press on with the attack while the good weather lasted. At the same time, he knew that if he failed he would receive all the blame. If he were to succeed, the credit would be given to Barron. Yet the difficulties were mounting. Drinking water was running short, as always in ships that carried their supplies in wooden barrels. Some of the water had been five months in the casks, in a hot climate. Even so, it was necessary to put an armed sentry over the water to prevent the thirsty men from drinking all they wanted.

In addition, scurvy was making its appearance among the men—the horrible disease that rotted men's jaws and covered their bodies with sores. Scurvy was to be expected in ships that had been long at sea with the men fed only on salted meat and dry biscuit. We know now that it is caused by the absence of Vitamin C. Preble was aware that fresh vegetables would cure it, and he had to turn aside from his task of planning the next attack to make arrangements to obtain vegetables along with fresh water.

A greater problem was that the ships themselves were wearing out as a result of continuous service. Ropes and canvas were becoming worn, in addition to the damage done by the enemy's fire. The *John Adams* had brought fresh supplies of needed goods, but they had to be transferred at sea, with the ships rolling and tossing in the stormy Mediterranean.

Preble faced his difficulties without flinching, re-equipped his ships, sent to Sicily for water and vegetables, and went in again and again to the attack. He tried everything that his active, clever mind could suggest. He made night attacks, for he knew that not only would the shore batteries find it harder to aim in the darkness, but the population would resent having to spend sleepless nights while the bomb vessels were at work. He pressed his attack on the Tripolitan gunboats until the American light craft actually came under the fire of musketry from the shore. He took the *Constitution* boldly into the harbor to pour her fire into the castle and the batteries.

As the days passed and the weather grew more and more unfavorable he resolved on one last desperate stroke. He would send an explosion ship into the harbor. She would be filled with tons of gunpowder. A brave crew would take her in at night, right up against the city, would light the fuses, and try to escape. (Preble knew that there would be no lack of volunteers for any venture, however dangerous.) The explosion would destroy the shipping sheltering under the castle, and with luck would wreck the castle and unroof every house.

The vessel selected for the attempt was one with a long history, the ketch *Intrepid*. She had already played the leading part in one of the most glorious episodes in the campaign—the burning of the *Philadelphia*. Now she was to make another daring entrance into the Tripoli harbor.

Master-Commandant Richard Somers volunteered for the command. He was an old friend of Decatur's, and had been at school with him in Philadelphia. However, the fortunes of war and accidents of weather had prevented him from covering himself with glory as Decatur had succeeded in doing. Other officers and men volunteered for the service; more than one man contrived to get on board in defiance of orders.

Seven tons of gunpowder were jammed into the hold of the little vessel. Then to increase the violence of the explosion and to scatter further destruction, heaps of shells, scrap iron, and solid shot were placed on top of the gunpowder. There were masses of combustibles which the explosion might send, flaming, into the enemy's ships and magazines. After the powder trains were laid, the fuses were put into position.

At nine o'clock in the evening of September 4th, when it was pitch dark and a gentle wind was blowing conveniently into the harbor, the *Intrepid* was ready for action. Somers, Lieutenant Henry Wadsworth, his second in command, Lieutenant Joseph Israel, an officer who came without orders, and the ten or more brave men of his crew, took the ship in through the darkness. Her escort saw her go; then they saw the orange flashes of the Tripolitan guns piercing the night as they opened fire on the *Intrepid*.

Those aboard her escort had every hope that the *Intrepid* would be able to make her way through gunfire directed by men who were taken by surprise and blinded by their own gun flashes. But the hope was baseless, and the heroism and self-sacrifice of the thirteen volunteers were wasted. Something went wrong. Perhaps she was hit by a shot from the batteries. Perhaps a man—perhaps Somers himself—waiting with a light in his hand was hit and fell. Perhaps there was an accident, as well there might be in a ship full of explosives on a desperate mission and under hostile fire.

The watchers saw a great flash, too soon, far too soon, for the *Intrepid* to have reached her goal. The flash lit up the spars and rigging that were flung high into the air.

There was a fountain of exploding shells, and then there was darkness and silence. The thirteen men were dead. The *Intrepid* had blown up when she was barely through the gap in the reef, and the damage she had done to Tripoli was negligible.

Perhaps, some might say, it would have been better if the attempt had never been made, for the Tripolitans were emboldened by the knowledge that the Americans, for all their courage and ingenuity, had failed. Now the Tripolitans could await further attacks with a confidence that had been considerably weakened by the previous assaults.

Preble was of a mind to show them their error. The very day after the *Intrepid* exploded he ordered a fresh attack, but the weather turned unkind as usual, so the attack had to be called off. And the weather showed no signs of relenting. The unhandy gunboats and mortar vessels would be in grave danger on that rocky coast. Ammunition—especially after seven tons of gunpowder had been lost in the *Intrepid*—was running short. Men and material were wearing out. Preble had to decide to return to the old system of blockade, and he sent his light craft back to Sicily.

No sooner had he done so than Commodore Barron arrived at last with the frigates and the stores that would have been so useful a month earlier. There was no place for Preble in the new squadron. Already a sick man, he handed over his command, to the sorrow of everyone who had served under him. Before leaving, he gave Barron what help he could in maintaining good relations with the British at Malta and Gibraltar and with the Sicilians at Palermo and Syracuse. Then he sailed for home. Preble had not long to live; not long enough to see the officers he had trained attain the glory and distinction which was to be theirs in later years. It was under Preble that Decatur and Macdonough and many others acquired the habits of thought and the professional ability which won victories for them later on.

Preble (we know from his letters that he pronounced his name "Prebble") can be looked upon as the man who made the most important contribution to the founding of the United States Navy. He was hot-tempered and severe, but his subordinates loved him. He left the Mediterranean with Tripoli still a source of trouble, but he had trained an efficient navy. The example he set, customs he established, and the tradition that he began were to last long after his death. His genius for organization and his grasp of naval problems left their mark on all the subsequent history of the United States.

# CHAPTER 9

# JEFFERSON CONSIDERS LANDING TROOPS IN NORTH AFRICA

AFTER PREBLE'S DEPARTURE, BARRON TOOK over the task of reducing Tripoli to reason. Winter with its gales was close at hand; there could be no question of further attacks on the port, but the blockade could be maintained vigorously. There were repeated captures and several skirmishes when blockade runners tried to take refuge on the coast under the protection of the Tripolitan army.

It should always be remembered what those brief and seemingly insignificant words imply, that "the blockade could be maintained vigorously." It meant that the officers and men suffered endless hardship, in little wooden ships heaving and rolling on stormy seas, their days filled with hard work and dull discomfort.

Those ships always leaked in bad weather, both below the water line and above, for the seams worked with the motion of the ship, opening and shutting as the ship strained on the waves. Every day there would be dreary hours of work on the pumps. Bedding and clothing would always be a little damp.

At any hour of the day or night the watch on deck, and sometimes all hands, would be called upon to hurry aloft to shorten sail or to make more sail. They would clamber about, a hundred feet above the deck, in lashing rain and often in pitch darkness for an hour or two of exhausting labor.

The damp hammocks to which the men could return to rest were crowded together. In the big spar-decked frigates the men could consider themselves lucky; each could sling his hammock in a space fully thirty inches wide, under a deck nearly six feet high. In the brigs and schooners the crowding was much worse—the men might be restricted to a space less than two feet wide for each hammock, under a deck no more than five feet six inches high. They might actually sling their hammocks in two layers; the least lifting of the head when lying there meant bumping it on the man above, or the deck above, according to which layer one happened to be lying in.

Overhead the hatches would be closed tight to keep out the sea that broke over the deck, and the packed mass of humanity below would swing, all together, with the movement of the ship. The smell of the stores and the bilge water would come up from below, and the rats would scurry about, their squeaks plainly to be heard above the snoring of the men and the groaning of the woodwork.

The seamen faced months of this life at a time, with only salted food to sustain them, and the officers were hardly better off. They were nearly as cramped and crowded, nearly as damp as the crews. Then too, they had the responsibility of keeping the ship off the rocks and shoals of one of the most dangerous coasts in the world. They had to hold her in a position from which she could cut off the blockade runners that sneaked among the shoals during good weather.

A commander needed a resolute mind to subject himself and his men to these hardships, especially when it was easy to think up some excuse to return to the peace and comfort of the harbors of Malta or Syracuse. It was hardly to be wondered at that, at the end of that winter, 1804–05, Commodore Barron found his health giving way, so that he had to turn over the command to Captain John Rodgers—the fifth commander-in-chief in four years.

Rodgers in his turn took on the duty of forcing the stubborn Tripolitans to sue for peace. But during that winter a fresh enterprise had been set in motion which might bring the war to an end. It is interesting to note that until this time, after four years of war, President Jefferson, although he was a brilliant man, had not come to appreciate one of the necessary factors in the employment of sea power.

Command of the sea implies a great deal. The power

that commands the sea can send its ships where it wishes, and it can prevent the weaker power from sending its ships to sea at all—in each case, of course, subject to the few exceptions of raiders and blockade runners. The stronger power can gradually wear down its enemy by compelling the weaker power to use up its resources. Jefferson saw this clearly enough. But nearly always sea power, to make itself fully felt, needs the help of military force. In 1945, when the American Navy had won the command of the sea from the Japanese, the capture of Okinawa by the American 10th Army enormously increased the pressure that would be brought to bear on Japan both by sea and air.

And thanks to sea power, the military force need not be very large. Sea power can transport an army quickly and secretly, to strike at any point. The power which is weaker at sea cannot guard against these blows very effectively. During World War II Japan had many more than a million men available whom she would gladly have employed at Okinawa if the American Navy had allowed her to.

In the same way, an army could have been profitably used against Tripoli. The moment the war began America should have dispatched a small army to North Africa. Only from five to ten thousand men would have been needed to defeat the Tripolitan army in battle. Landing an American army on the rugged African coast near enough to make a prompt attack on the city would have been difficult, but it could have been done.

Siege artillery would have been needed to breach the walls of the city ready for the troops to assault, but that would not have been hard to provide. Probably it would never have had to be employed. If when Dale first arrived off Tripoli, the Tripolitans had heard that he had ten thousand men and a siege train ready to land, the Tripolitans would have surrendered instantly. They would have agreed to any terms whatever, sooner than endure an attack.

But that was only a dream. There was no chance of Congress in 1801 authorizing the raising of an army of even four thousand men or of agreeing to its dispatch overseas. In those days the whole American army was numbered by the hundreds, not by the thousands. Even so, it was looked upon with great suspicion as a weapon that might some day be used by a tyrant.

It would have been impossible to persuade either Jefferson or Congress that sending out an army with Dale would be cheaper in the end. Didn't everyone expect that Dale would force peace on Tripoli by means of his unaided naval force in a single summer? No one in 1801 believed for a moment that in 1805 America would still be hurriedly building ships and sending them out to continue the war that was so lightheartedly entered upon.

It should also be borne in mind that sending an army overseas is not a business to be lightly undertaken. It calls for much planning and much experience. To transport an army capable of dealing with Tripoli would have needed a fleet of at least a hundred transports, which America could only have collected with difficulty at that time. To keep men and horses in health during a long sea voyage was a hard matter, and to make sure they had every necessity for warfare with them needed much experience.

Then, too, there was always the chance that the army, even when landed, might be wiped out by disease, as England had discovered more than once.

Brilliantly successful landings, like those of General Eisenhower in North Africa in 1942 and in Normandy in 1944, have to be worked for as well as hoped for. They cannot be taken for granted. The Federal government, at the time of the blockade of Tripoli, did not have the necessary staff to direct and organize an amphibious expedition on any scale, small or large.

CHAPTER 10

# EATON ATTACKS BY LAND
# ACROSS DESERT

IN SPITE OF THE STRONG FEELING AGAINST
an army, the idea of striking at Tripoli by a land force
supported by the Navy had long been in existence.
William Eaton (he usually called himself "general" but
the American government was always careful to speak of
him as "Mr.") had been United States consul in North
Africa for a considerable time. His appointment dated
back to 1797, and he had been there off and on since 1799.
During that time he had acquired a good deal of experience of North African politics. He was a busy, active man;
the suggestions he pressed upon Dale and Morris were

among the distractions those unfortunate men had to contend with.

Eaton had ideas about the employment of a land force. So had James L. Cathcart, who had an even more intimate knowledge of North Africa, because he had been a prisoner in Algiers for ten years. There he had become secretary to the Dey (thanks to his knowledge of languages), and from 1799 had been United States consul in Tripoli. Cathcart and Eaton had done much to stir up enemies against Tripoli. They had played a part in the negotiations which had opened the ports of Naples to the American Navy and which had secured the help of the Neapolitan gunboats. Cathcart and Eaton had also hoped at times to secure the services of a Neapolitan army. They were both aware of the existence of a man who might be employed to bring pressure on the Pasha of Tripoli.

This man was Hamet, who might be described as a prince of the royal house of Tripoli. His father had been the bloodthirsty Ali Karamanli, who had managed to maintain himself as Pasha for thirty years, and even to die a natural death in the end.

After Ali's death in 1796, his youngest son, Yusuf, had seized the throne. Yusuf caught one of his elder brothers and murdered him. Another brother, Hamet, managed to escape to Tunis, where he stayed for some time. This worried Yusuf, who was always afraid that Hamet might be used as a figurehead for a rebellion against him. Yusuf made tempting offers to try to get Hamet into his clutches, but Hamet was too cautious.

In the end Yusuf—when the American fleet was in the Mediterranean—offered his brother Hamet a magnificent bribe, nothing less than the half of his kingdom. He appointed Hamet governor of Derna, the chief town of the eastern part of the state. No one can doubt that the offer was made in the hope that sooner or later Hamet would come within Yusuf's reach.

Having been turned out of Tunis, Hamet accepted the offer for he was at his wits' end regarding how to support himself. Then he carefully sailed direct from Malta to Derna without risking an interview with his terrible brother. The odd situation lasted for nearly a year, and then Hamet, quite certain that Yusuf was still scheming for his murder, attempted to rebel, was defeated, and only just escaped with his life. He went to Egypt, and there once more faced the problem of how to get enough to eat.

Eaton and Cathcart had long had their eye on Hamet. The golden opportunity had passed, which was when he was actually in rebellion at Derna. At that time Eaton was in the United States, pressing his scheme upon the administration. By the time President Jefferson and Secretary of the Navy Smith were convinced of the advantages to be gained by supporting Hamet, he had been appointed governor, had rebelled, and had fled to Egypt. However, this news had not yet reached America. Mr. Madison, as Secretary of State, was at last persuaded it was not "unfair" (that was his own word) to support Hamet against his bloodthirsty and black-mailing brother.

So Eaton returned to the Mediterranean in the spring of 1804, empowered to arrange to act in concert with Hamet. And Rodgers received orders to listen to Eaton's advice on how to use Hamet to the best advantage. It was

131

a little upsetting to find that Hamet had disappeared and had abandoned his government of Derna. Still, Eaton was not going to lose the chance of carrying out a plan he had advocated for the past two years and for which he had already crossed the Atlantic twice. His instructions from the Secretary of the Navy had their effect on Barron (this was before Barron relinquished his command to Rodgers). Isaac Hull, Master and Commandant, with his brig *Argus,* was detailed to help Eaton find Hamet and then to assist in any land campaign that might be waged.

Off went Eaton, aboard the *Argus,* to Alexandria. He found Egypt at the time in a state of complete disorder. The Turks were trying to reconquer the country. The Mamelukes—a gang of military chiefs who had ruled Egypt for centuries before Napoleon's conquest of the country seven years before—were trying to regain their power. Various other officers and officials were trying to establish themselves as independent chieftains. War and disease, famine and poverty, rebellion and treachery, had set the whole country in a turmoil.

The British diplomats present were helpful and reliable. On the other hand, the French diplomats, because France was at war with England, thought it their duty to try to balk every British effort. This was done even though England was trying to subdue Tripoli.

But by the aid of the British diplomats, Eaton succeeded in locating Hamet and eventually in getting into communication with him. He was found to be with the Mameluke army far in the interior.

Persuading Hamet to try to become Pasha of Tripoli was a hard task. The wretched man was afraid that the whole scheme was a plan of his brother's to get him into his power and strangle him. Even if it was not as bad as that, Hamet was still afraid that the Americans might hand him over to Yusuf. His fears for his life made him nervous and difficult to deal with. At one point he even ran away for refuge into the desert. But in the end Eaton persuaded Hamet to meet him in a personal conference, and at that conference persuaded him to join in the attempt.

Eaton was determined that the attempt should be made. He was so set upon it that he made promises in the name of the United States that he had no power to make. The final agreement included the shameful clause that Hamet should repay the United States (when at last he should be ruler of Tripoli) out of the money he would extort from other countries. There was apparently no thought in Eaton's mind of putting an end to the whole disgraceful system of piracy and blackmail.

With the agreement signed, Eaton set about the task of raising an army. This should not have been a very difficult task in Egypt where troops without leaders roamed everywhere, but Eaton had very little money. What he had started out with had already been sadly reduced by the need for bribing Turkish officials.

Eaton afterwards declared that with money he could have raised an army of twenty thousand men, and he was probably right. But as it was, he could only offer promises. He might attract troops of a sort by the promise of a share in the plunder of Tripoli, but to obtain food and weapons and ammunition in that famine-ridden country he needed cash. So it was that Eaton exhausted all his resources in scraping together a few stores.

Yet an army was assembled, if it can be called such. It was made up of Moors and Arabs and Greeks, wild Bedouin chieftains, and some stray Austrian and Italian adventurers. There must have been many moments during the expedition when Eaton felt glad that he had with him a personal bodyguard of seven Marines with Lieutenant Presley O'Bannon and Midshipman Pascal Peck. They were the only trustworthy individuals in the whole force of four hundred men.

The tiny army was gathered in the dreary desert overlooking the sea, not far from a place whose name would not be famous for another hundred and forty years—El Alamein. The *Argus* was sent off to Malta with an appeal from Eaton to Barron for food and weapons and money. Then the mob started on their five-hundred-mile march through the country where so much later Rommel and Montgomery, Germans and British and Italians, were to march and suffer in the African campaigns of World War II.

Eaton's force suffered terribly from hunger and thirst as they struggled along, and it was only natural that discouragement and faint-heartedness should make their appearance. Every man knew that in the event of defeat the best he could hope for was slavery, and at worst he would suffer death by torture.

Hamet himself had never had much enthusiasm for the project. The promises Eaton made lost their appeal to men who were hungry and weary. Eaton faced several mutinies. He had to persuade Hamet against abandoning the expedition and retiring to a quieter life in Egypt.

It is quite amazing that Eaton succeeded in keeping the expedition moving forward even slowly—he must have been a man of most persuasive tongue. There was one occasion when by the slaughter of a camel and sheep he was able to provide what he called a "full ration" for his four hundred men. He must have talked very glibly to have persuaded the four hundred into agreeing with him.

For five weeks Eaton coaxed his army along over the five hundred miles of desert. He even tried to drill them into discipline and order as they marched.

At last they struggled into Bomba, a desolate bay without houses or people. And there, in the nick of time, arrived the *Argus,* to keep the appointment made weeks before. From the *Argus,* and from the *Hornet* next day, Eaton received food and ammunition and, equally important, seven thousand dollars in cash.

It was equally important, but disappointing, that the *Argus* and the *Hornet* could spare Eaton no reinforcement in men. There were no marines available, and the little ships had only enough trained seamen for their own purposes, with none to spare for adventures on land. Eaton would have to make do with what he had.

The whole incident was a striking example of the influence of sea power. Without the promise of ships to meet them, Eaton would never have been able to induce his army to move in the first place. And if by some evil chance Yusuf in Tripoli had been able to regain command of the sea and chase away the American squadron, Eaton and his men would have suffered death in the desert or slavery.

With his army fed and paid, Eaton should have had no difficulty in leading it forward over the remaining sixty miles to Derna. But that did not come to pass. Rumors that the army of Tripoli was on the march for Derna sent the whole force into a panic. The men were terrified of Yusuf's cruelty, and wanted to retreat out of harm's way. By some means, Eaton persuaded them to move forward, and three more days of marching brought the four hundred up to the fortifications of Derna.

The sea front and the eastern side of Derna that faced Eaton's army had been fortified, but not very well. Eaton looked the situation over, and sent in a demand for surrender. This was refused, although people inside the town who wanted to make sure of being on the winning side, no matter who won, sent out messages saying they hoped for Eaton's victory.

There was no time to waste. With the passage of time Eaton's army might melt away and Yusuf's army might arrive. Eaton recognized the fact, and he was a man of energy and resolution.

During this time the *Argus* and *Hornet* were anchored off the town, as had been agreed. Now the little *Nautilus*, with her shallow draft and handy rig, was at hand as well.

Eaton needed artillery to batter the defenses; the squadron had a couple of field guns for him. They were landed on the beach, but above the beach rose a steep cliff. One gun was dragged up by main force, and with a single gun at his disposal Eaton would not delay another minute. He had the gun dragged to a little hilltop and set his Greek gunners to work firing on the fortifications.

At the same time, the *Argus* and the *Hornet* and the *Nautilus* came creeping into the shallows as far as they dared, and opened a steady fire on the waterfront. The enemy blazed away in return, bullets flying and some men dropping.

In the excitement one of Eaton's gunners fired off the gun before the ramrod had been withdrawn after ramming down the shot. The ramrod went sailing off toward the enemy's line. It was quite a sight, no doubt, but it meant that the gun was now useless, and its resounding bang would no longer be heard to encourage Eaton's men and dishearten the enemy. With the gun rendered useless, there was no time to lose. Eaton, who had kept his head clear and his spirits high, called on his men to charge. Forward they went, the handful of marines leading, the Greeks behind them, and the Arabs cautiously following up. Fortunately they were faced by an enemy as undisciplined and as shaky as themselves.

The bold attack turned the scale, as Eaton, much to his credit, had realized was to be expected. The garrison fled, but here and there a man turned back to empty his loaded musket at the attackers. One bullet shattered Eaton's wrist, just too late for it to have any effect on the battle.

Lieutenant O'Bannon and Midshipman George Mann knew the importance of keeping a beaten enemy on the run, and they kept the attack moving. Battery and guns were captured, and the guns were turned on the defenders when they tried to rally in the fortified houses. They fled again, and in a few wild minutes the battle was over. Eaton's army held the town, and the wretched Hamet, still much worried about his future, was installed in the governor's palace.

A price had to be paid for victory. Of the seven gallant marines who had followed O'Bannon and formed the spearhead of the attack, two were dead and one was wounded. In addition, Eaton and several Greeks were wounded.

The crisis was not yet over. Most of the garrison of Derna, having fled from the town, assembled again outside it. And Eaton's boldness and promptness in capturing the town was thoroughly justified by the arrival, scarcely more than a week later, of the Tripolitan army.

Despite his wound, Eaton had to work hard to keep his army fighting. There were numerous skirmishes as the Tripolitans circled about the town and risked timid attacks; but Eaton had the guns of the fortifications at his disposal now. And once or twice the *Argus,* searching along the coast, caught parties of the enemy within range and sent cannon balls into them.

Unlike Eaton, the Tripolitan commander could not inspire his men to risk all in a headlong attack. As a result, Eaton was able to hold on to his conquest, and the

Tripolitan army was faced with the necessity of trying to maintain itself in the desert. No doubt it would have speedily melted away—Eaton thought (and he was probably right) that with a little money he could have induced the whole Tripolitan force to come over to his side—if fresh news had not come from Tripoli at that moment.

# CHAPTER 11

# PIRATES SUBDUED — PEACE REIGNS ON THE HIGH SEAS AT LAST

PEACE WAS MADE. THE BLOCKADE OF TRIPOLI had been maintained, and prizes had been taken. Reinforcements were still arriving from America, and more were expected. These included gunboats which were American built and American manned and which could be used in a fresh attack on the port. One of these tiny craft was lost with all hands crossing the Atlantic but seven others succeeded in making the passage.

The Tripolitans were growing disheartened, and now they were faced by the appalling threat of an attack by land. They weighed the fact that Eaton had made the fantastic march from Egypt to Derna. What was there to prevent his making the no more fantastic march from Derna to Tripoli? If ships could be collected to transport him by sea he might be at the gates of Tripoli within a week.

Thus ran the Tripolitans' thoughts, for in times of war neither side realizes how serious are the other side's difficulties. So Yusuf was anxious to make peace, and he found to his pleased surprise that the Americans with whom he was dealing were equally anxious. They were not determined on his abdication, or on his death, or on the destruction of the fortifications of Tripoli. It actually seemed as if they would be satisfied with promises. And promises cost nothing.

Within a day or two of the beginning of the new bargaining, Yusuf ceased to look over his shoulder at the fearful menace of his brother's advance on Derna. Yusuf's only problem now was finding out how much the Americans would give him.

Tobias Lear, who had the duty of conducting the

bargaining on the American side, had been George Washington's private secretary. Since 1803, Lear had held the position of Consul General, and was anxious to make a name for himself as a diplomat. It was a temptation to think of himself as the man who made peace when everyone before him had failed. More than once he had pressed upon Preble the acceptance of terms which Preble thought ridiculous. Now he had complete control over the negotiations, for Barron was very ill—more than one letter hints that he was not quite sane.

Lear had the advantage of knowing that he had the support of every man in the American naval force outside Tripoli. They were worried about the three hundred prisoners whom Yusuf had held captive for eighteen months. Any agreement that would set them free had merit in the eyes of their comrades. It was a difficult question.

In war the decision of an officer, often comfortably out of danger, may send other men to their deaths. The public that agrees to war, or that demands war, is demanding at the same time that men should be killed. Many people

145

do not consider that unpleasant fact because they do not know which men shall die.

It is a harder thing to decide that a group of men, whose names are known, shall continue to suffer hardship and captivity, when a word may set them free. That word may cost lives in the future; it may abandon to the enemy what other men have died for, but it is hard not to say it.

The prisoners were not suffering as badly in their confinement as they might have suffered. That is not saying a great deal, for the man who has lost his liberty has lost almost everything already. The enlisted men's hardships were lessened by the generous expenditures of money, by the efforts of the foreign consuls, and by the devoted work of Jonathan Cowdery, the surgeon's mate, and Jacob Jones, the second lieutenant. Six of the three hundred men died. This is a small number when it is remembered that they spent eighteen months in an unsanitary city that had a high death rate.

No officer died; and the officers had some small compensation for the loss of a year and a half out of their young lives. This was brought about by their attendance at what David Porter called the University of the Prison: the classes that Porter started with the aid of textbooks supplied by the Danish consul. Every officer had something to teach, and everyone had much to learn; mathematics and navigation, languages and tactics and seamanship. There were classes in all these subjects and the young men learned much about the theory of their profession.

Daniel Patterson and James Biddle are only two among the many distinguished names of the graduates of Tripoli University, although it can never be doubted that any one of the prisoners would gladly have given all his learning in exchange for liberty. Nor can it be doubted that the chances of peace being made and the chances of being set free were discussed far more frequently than the rules of grammar.

So peace was made. The Tripolitans gave their promises. They promised peace and good behavior. They promised that if by misfortune they should ever again be at war with the United States (despite the other promise), they would agree to an exchange of prisoners and would never again ask for ransom. But this time, just this once, they wanted ransom money, and Lear yielded the point. To liberate the ship's company of the *Philadelphia,* Lear handed over sixty thousand dollars and eighty-nine prisoners.

The Tripolitans were most obliging. They accepted the American promise and actually set free Bainbridge and his men before the arrival of the ransom money. They saluted the Stars and Stripes. The Pasha—the unspeakable Yusuf—gave Lear an audience in his palace.

At the same time the treaty made it inevitable that Hamet and his men, whom Eaton had coaxed from Egypt to Derna, should be abandoned. Eaton succeeded in carrying off by sea Hamet and some of his friends. All the rest of the four hundred, and all the inhabitants of Derna who had been unwise enough to declare for Hamet, were left behind.

There was a promise from Yusuf that he would take no action against these people, but in Derna no one believed Yusuf's promises. At the moment when the rejoicing prisoners were being set free in Tripoli, there was despair in Derna. There was violence, too, and Eaton only succeeded in getting himself and Hamet into the ships under cover of his artillery. When he left the place, the people he left behind were preparing for flight into the desert. They were willing to undergo the awful hardships of the six-hundred-mile track to Egypt rather than trust to Yusuf's promises. Eaton had made them promises as well, and no doubt he had not been empowered by his government to make those promises, but it was a pity.

We do not know what happened in Derna when Yusuf's army marched in, but we hear occasional news of Hamet afterwards. We find Hamet and his fifteen followers living in Syracuse on two hundred dollars a month allowed him by Rodgers. We find Hamet petitioning the President for help, and being awarded twenty-four hundred dollars, which took a year to arrive.

Then came the discovery that Lear had secretly agreed to allow Yusuf to keep Hamet's wife and children for four years as hostages. America exerted herself then to persuade Yusuf to hand them over and provide Hamet with a pension. Next we find Hamet actually reinstated as governor of Derna (no one can ever guess what will happen next when a tyrant rules). Finally Hamet fled away to Egypt again and we hear no more of him.

Yusuf lived on for many years in the verminous splendor of his palace in Tripoli. The man who could outface and outbargain the United States was cunning enough and resolute enough to deal with rebellious soldiers and treacherous admirals.

On the edge of the ebb and flow of the world war that engulfed Europe and eventually involved America, Tripoli lay in a comfortable eddy and no power was able to spare ships or army to keep her in order. Yusuf profited as a neutral, and he profited as an occasional belligerent. Privateers who were not too sure of the legality of their captures sold their prizes to him.

He also speculated with profit in the wartime markets, and he did not cling fervently to his neutrality when confronted by a superior force. In the stress of the War of 1812, the Stars and Stripes disappeared from the Mediterranean save when displayed by an occasional privateer. To reword an old proverb, when honest men fell out rogues made the most of their opportunity.

Then suddenly and dramatically the situation changed. The wars ended, and the enormous fleets which for years had fought each other were now free to punish the Barbary States. The Treaty of Ghent had barely been signed before America decided to deal with the Mediterranean nuisance.

America was elated with the victories won at sea during the war with England. She had a navy that had grown up on the solid foundation laid by Preble, a navy that knew its own worth, commanded by men who had passed the test of war. Mr. Madison and Congress were both ready to fight to maintain the dignity of their country. The ships were ready and the men were ready, and experience had shown the value of time.

A squadron sailed in the spring of 1815. Eleven years after Decatur had crept into Tripoli in the little *Intrepid*, he appeared in the Mediterranean in command of a large force. The list of his ships included the glorious names of the *Macedonian* and the *Guerrière*.

The rapidity of Decatur's movements took the world—especially the pirate world—by surprise. Less than a month after he sailed from New York, the flagship of Algiers was a prize and the Algerine admiral was dead on his own quarterdeck. Five weeks after sailing, Decatur was in Algiers harbor dictating terms of peace.

He then took on fresh water and provisions, and within a month was entering Tunis. Tunis could make no defense, and the world was treated to the extraordinary spectacle of a Barbary State handing over hard cash in payment of reparations for breaches of neutrality. No time was wasted; Tunis yielded and paid up in a week.

In three days more Decatur was off Tripoli, bringing with him the news of what had happened in Tunis and hard on the heels of the news of what had happened in Algiers.

From the quarterdeck of the *Guerrière,* Decatur could look over at the castle and the minarets, at the long reef where he had fought for his life with cutlass against pike, at the harbor where he had won his promotion by burning the *Philadelphia*. And Yusuf could look out from his palace and see the American ships, cleared for action, and meditate on the fact that they were commanded by a man who meant business.

Yet in this, our last sight of Yusuf, we have to accord him some amused respect. He knew he had to yield, but of all the North African rulers he alone succeeded in bargaining with Decatur in the face of all Decatur's guns. Thirty thousand dollars was the sum Decatur demanded in damages; but Yusuf beat him down to twenty-five thousand, and finally clinched the bargain by throwing in a thousand dollars' worth of slaves. We can hardly wonder that Yusuf lived on for many years after that; the man who could get the better of a bargain with Decatur in all the flush of victory was a man capable of dealing with most problems.

But even so, Yusuf tasted humiliation and defeat, with a rapidity that could hardly be believed. Less than six months after Congress had declared war, the bags of gold were being ferried out to the *Guerrière* in Tripoli. The American flag was safe from insult, and American citizens were safe from outrage.

# Index

# ABOUT THE AUTHOR

C. S. Forester was born in Cairo, Egypt in 1899. He was educated in England and considered becoming a doctor, but soon became more interested in writing novels. Forester was thirty-six when his most famous book, *The African Queen,* appeared. Later this story became a classic film starring Humphrey Bogart and Katharine Hepburn.

Forester's best-known books are sea stories. His depictions of life at sea are vivid and filled with accurate nautical detail. Forester was on a freighter voyage when he created a most remarkable character—Horatio Hornblower, a swashbuckling hero and British naval officer during the period of the Napoleonic Wars. Forester gave his character many small weaknesses (he suffers from seasickness and is shy), and the public loved him and demanded more and more stories. Eventually there were eleven Hornblower novels plus a few short stories. Many of these were later produced for film and television.

In addition to his fiction work, C. S. Forester wrote *Nelson,* a biography, *The Age of Fighting Sail* and *The Naval War of 1812.*

# BOOKS IN THIS SERIES

# ✷STERLING POINT BOOKS

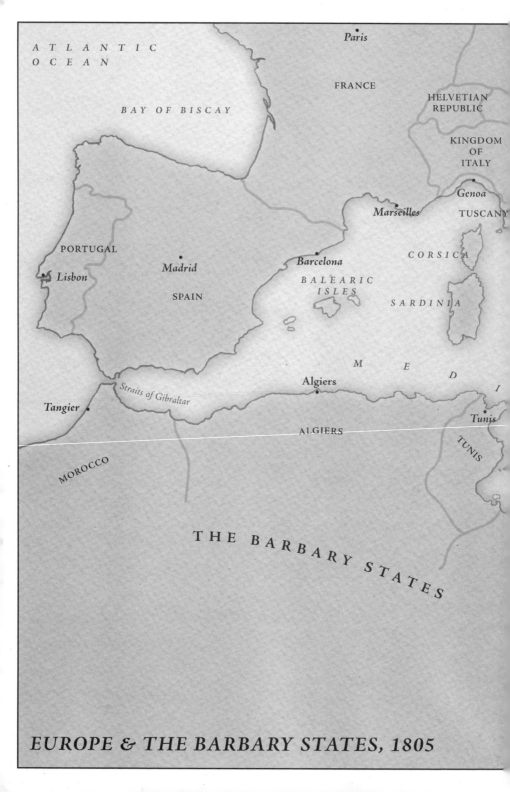

# EUROPE & THE BARBARY STATES, 1805